OXFORD MEDICAL PUBLICATIONS

Oxford Handbook of

Oral and Maxillofacial Surgery

Published and forthcoming Oxford Handbooks

Oxford Handbook of
Oral and Maxillofacial Surgery

Luke Cascarini

Consultant Oral and Maxillofacial Surgeon,
North West London Hospitals NHS Trust,
Honorary Consultant at The Royal Marsden
Hospital and West Middlesex
University Hospital, London, UK

Clare Schilling

Specialist Trainee in Oral and Maxillofacial Surgery,
London, UK

Ben Gurney

Specialist Trainee in Oral and Maxillofacial Surgery,
Guildford, UK

Peter Brennan

Consultant Oral and Maxillofacial Surgeon,
Queen Alexandra Hospital,
Portsmouth, UK

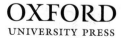

OXFORD
UNIVERSITY PRESS

OXFORD
UNIVERSITY PRESS

Great Clarendon Street, Oxford OX2 6DP

Oxford University Press is a department of the University of Oxford.
It furthers the University's objective of excellence in research, scholarship,
and education by publishing worldwide in

Oxford New York

Auckland Cape Town Dar es Salaam Hong Kong Karachi
Kuala Lumpur Madrid Melbourne Mexico City Nairobi
New Delhi Shanghai Taipei Toronto

With offices in

Argentina Austria Brazil Chile Czech Republic France Greece
Guatemala Hungary Italy Japan Poland Portugal Singapore
South Korea Switzerland Thailand Turkey Ukraine Vietnam

Oxford is a registered trade mark of Oxford University Press
in the UK and in certain other countries

Published in the United States
by Oxford University Press Inc., New York

British Library Cataloguing in Publication Data
Data available

Library of Congress Cataloging-in-Publication Data

Oxford handbook of oral and maxillofacial surgery / Luke Cascarini . . . [et al.].
    p. ; cm. — (Oxford handbooks)
Handbook of oral and maxillofacial surgery
Includes bibliographical references and index.
ISBN 978-0-19-958329-4 (alk. paper)
1. Mouth—Surgery--Handbooks, manuals, etc. 2. Face—Surgery—Handbooks, manuals, etc.
3. Maxilla—Surgery—Handbooks, manuals, etc. I. Cascarini, Luke. II. Title: Handbook of oral
and maxillofacial surgery. III. Series: Oxford handbooks.
[DNLM: 1. Oral Surgical Procedures—Handbooks. WU 49]
RK529.O94 2011
617.5'22059—dc23   2011027609

Typeset by Cenveo, Bangalore, India
Printed in China
on acid-free paper through
Asia Pacific Offset

ISBN 978–0–19–958329–4

10 9 8 7 6 5 4 3 2 1

Foreword

The trainee entering the exciting field of oral and maxillofacial surgery has every reason to feel rather nervous. Not only is he or she confronted by large number of patients with all sorts of interesting, difficult, complex, and confusing problems – some of which may be outside the strict boundaries of the head and neck – but also by the bewildering number of large, beautifully illustrated, and very expensive textbooks which are available on the subject. Fortunately, to the rescue come the four authors of this book; two of them experienced surgical teachers in this field, reinforced by two specialist trainees in oral and maxillofacial surgery. They have succeeded in producing a concise aid, which covers pretty well all the problems the tyro is likely to encounter in everyday clinical practice; the specialized anatomy and radiology of the region, what to do on the wards, the clinics, the theatre and the A and E department, how to cope with the drugs in common use and even how to get on with colleagues.

Although not a maxillofacial surgeon myself, I have read through this book with great interest. I am sure the trainees in this exciting and expanding speciality will benefit from using it – and so will their patients!

Harold Ellis CBE, FRCS.
Emeritus Professor of Surgery, University of London.

Preface

This book has been written to be your friend and guide during your time working as a doctor in oral and maxillofacial surgery. It has been written much like a travel guide, to give you the information you need when you need it. While it is full of factual information, it is not intended to be a concise textbook of oral and maxillofacial surgery (OMFS)—there are plenty of those available.

This book will tell you those things that other books won't! Really useful tips that we learned 'on the job' have been gathered and added to these pages, alongside practical hints and guidance. We have also included things you will feel you really should know but are afraid to ask.

A good book is a living thing. We have grown this book to its current stage over 18 months, and we sincerely hope that, as with other Oxford Handbooks, you will feed your own ideas and advice to us and it will continue to grow and evolve and thereby serve many generations of junior doctors in OMFS to come.

Good luck with your job and remember—it's a bad day when you haven't learned something new!

Luke Cascarini
Clare Schilling
Ben Gurney
Peter Brennan

Contents

Detailed contents

Symbols and abbreviations

Some of these are included because they are in common usage, others because they are long words and we were trying to save space.

📖	cross-reference
♂:♀	male: female ratio
▶	this is important
↑	increased
↓	decreased
<	lesser than
>	greater than
~	approximately
μ	micro (e.g. μg, μm)
A&E	accident and emergency
ACE	angiotensin-converting enzyme
AIDS	acquired immune deficiency syndrome
ALS	advanced life support
AOT	adenomatoid odontogenic tumour
AP	antero-posterior
ATLS	advanced trauma life support
AUG	acute ulcerative gingivitis
BAOMS	British Association of Oral and Maxillofacial Surgeons
BCC	basal cell carcinoma
bd	twice daily
BDA	British Dental Association
BMA	British Medical Association
BP	blood pressure
BRONJ	bisphosphonate related osteonecrosis of the jaw
BSV	binocular single vision
Ca^{2+}	calcium ion
CABG	coronary artery bypass graft
CAD/CAM	computer-aided design/computer-aided manufacturing
CEOT	calcifying epithelial odontogenic tumour
cm	centimetre
CMV	cytomegalovirus
CNS	central nervous system
CRP	C-reactive protein

CSF	cerebrospinal fluid
CT	computed tomography
CTA	CT angiography
CVA	cerebrovascular accident
CXR	chest X-ray
DCIA	deep circumflex iliac artery
DPT	dental panoramic tomogram (OPT/OPG)
DVT	deep vein thrombosis
EBV	Epstein–Barr virus
EM	erythema multiforme
ENT	ear, nose, and throat
ESR	erythrocyte sedimentation rate
EUA	examination under anaesthesia
FBC	full blood count
FNAC	fine-needle aspiration cytology
FOM	floor of mouth
g	gram
G&S	group and save
GA	general anaesthesia
GDC	General Dental Council
GDP	general dental practitioner
GI	gastrointestinal
GMC	General Medical Council
GMP	general medical practitioner
Hb	haemoglobin
HDU	high dependency unit
HIV	human immunodeficiency virus
HLA	human leucocyte antigen
HPV	human papilloma virus
HSV	herpes simplex virus
IAN	inferior alveolar nerve
ICU	intensive care unit
IDB	inferior dental block
IDN	inferior dental nerve
IMF	intermaxillary fixation
INR	International Normalized Ratio
ITP	idiopathic thrombocytopenic purpura
ITU	intensive therapy unit
IU	international units
IV	intravenous

LDH	lactate dehydrogenase
LFT	liver function test
LMA	laryngeal mask airway
LP	lichen planus
MALT	mucosa-associated lymphoid tissue
MAP	mean arterial pressure
mcg	microgram
MDT	multidisciplinary team
MEN	multiple endocrine neoplasia
mg	milligram
MHz	megahertz
micromol	micromoles
min	minute
ml	millilitre
mm	millimetre
mmHg	millimetres of mercury
mmol	millimole
MRA	magnetic resonance angiography
MRI	magnetic resonance imaging
MUA	manipulation under anaesthesia
NAI	non-accidental injury
NBM	nil by mouth
NGT	nasogastric tube
OAF	oro-antral fistula
OCP	oral contraceptive pill
od	once daily
OH	oral hygiene
OMFS	oral and maxillofacial surgery
OM	occipitomental
ORIF	open reduction and internal fixation
ORN	osteoradionecrosis
OVD	occlusal vertical dimension
PA	Posteroanterior
PDL	periodontal ligament
PEG	percutaneous endoscopic gastrostomy
PET	positron emission tomography
PO	per orum (by mouth)
PPI	proton pump inhibitor
PR	per rectum
PSA	pleomorphic salivary adenoma

qds	four times daily
QoL	quality of life
RAS	recurrent aphthous stomatitis
RBC	red blood cell count
RBH	retrobulbar haemorrhage
RCT	root canal treatment/therapy
RIG	radiologically inserted gastrostomy
SALT	speech and language therapist
SAN	spinal accessory nerve
SCC	squamous cell carcinoma
SCM	sternoclastoid muscle
sec	second
SMAS	superficial muscular aponeuritic system
SMG	submandibular gland
SUNCT	short-lasting unilateral neuralgiform headache attacks with conjunctival injection and tearing
tds	three times daily
TFT	thyroid function test
TMJ	temporomandibular joint
TMPDS	temporomandibular pain dysfunction syndrome
TTO	'to take out' (prescriptions in hospital discharge summary)
US	ultrasound
WCC	white cell count
X-rays	either X-ray beam or radiographs
ZA	zygomatic arch
ZF	zygomatic-frontal

Chapter 1

Overview

Using this book

- This book has been primarily written for junior doctors working in OMFS. We hope that it will appeal to both junior medical and junior dental practitioners. We realize that the medical undergraduate curriculum contains very little exposure to OMFS, so we apologize in advance to our dentally qualified readers if some of the dentally based chapters appear very basic!

- We have deliberately tried to avoid writing a condensed surgical textbook and have tried to provide a practical hands-on' travel guide' for you in your time as a junior in OMFS.

- We have also avoided reproducing information which you will already have in the medical and surgical books that you already own.

- The 'clinical areas' chapters make up the backbone of this book. This concept is the result of our desire to give you what you really need to know when you really need it. For example, consider fractured mandibles—the information you need to know about patient management is different depending on whether you are seeing a patient in the accident and emergency department (A&E), in theatre, on the ward, or as an outpatient.

- There are other chapters on subjects that we consider basic but essential for getting the most out of a job in OMFS, so we have called these chapters 'basic knowledge'.

- There is a chapter on essential skills which is no substitute for practical teaching but should get you out of a corner, as will the emergencies chapter. We hope that you will have read these in advance of being called upon to enact them!

- Oral medicine is a vast subject and no attempt has been made to condense it into this handbook. Instead, we have tried to provide a mixture of basic knowledge and practical tips on how to manage the oral medicine patient.

- We encourage you to spend some time looking at oral and maxillofacial radiographs and images whenever possible with a senior colleague. The radiology chapter cannot teach you how to recognize pathology on images and is only intended to provide some broad general radiological knowledge to support your learning.

- The other chapters provide general help where we think you might need it. We believe that a book is an organic thing; we have enjoyed writing this first edition and with your input we hope that it will evolve with time.

- We hope that this book will be more of a knowledgeable friend and guide than just a list of facts. After all, you can access facts on the internet.

- Finally, we hope that you enjoy your time in our specialty and wish you the very best of luck whatever career you choose.

OMFS—the specialty

- OMFS is one of the nine surgical specialties recognized by the surgical colleges and is regulated by the General Medical Council (GMC).
- It is a unique specialty. In the UK, to be appointed as a consultant in OMFS you must not only be on the GMC specialist list but also possess a registrable dental degree. It is now not necessary to be on the General Dental Council (GDC) register, and many consultants choose not to be.
- The same requirements are stipulated throughout the European Union.
- The specialty has evolved greatly in the last 25 years.
- In times past, oral surgery was a popular dental specialty which dealt with diseases of the jaws and mouth. But during both World Wars, oral surgeons were called upon to manage some of the vast amounts of oral *and maxillofacial* trauma. Probably because of this, the oral surgeons saw that there was a need for oral and maxillofacial specialists and the specialty grew. Our forefathers realized the need to have a proper medical education and surgical training, and so medical degrees became obligatory. Eventually the specialty ceased to be regulated by the GDC.
- This move left dentistry without an oral surgery specialist list and that void was filled. There is now a dental specialty, oral surgery, which is mainly confined to dental schools. Training pathways in oral surgery are now also starting to appear in district general hospitals.
- Some OMFS surgeons have become super-specialized and dropped the oral surgery component completely, and are dedicated craniofacial or head and neck cancer surgeons.
- However, most OMFS units manage the full remit of oral *and* maxillofacial surgery. While OMF surgeons have their historical roots in dentistry and hold their dental colleagues in the highest regard, OMFS has come a long way. OMF surgeons have the same basic surgical training as any other surgeon and additionally are trained in dentistry. Some have gone on to do higher research degrees. Most will not much appreciate being called a dentist!

Legal aspects of OMFS

If you have either GMC or GDC registration, you can work as a junior trainee in OMFS. To progress into higher surgical training in OMFS, dual qualification is required. Professional registration is now only required with the GMC as OMFS is classified as a medical rather than a dental specialty, although some surgeons are still registered with the GDC as well.

However, much of the clinical day-to-day workload in OMFS relates to the surgical aspects of dentistry. For example, the extraction, manipulation, or implantation of teeth could all be seen to fall within 'the practice of dentistry', although these are all relevant duties for an OMFS junior to undertake. Juniors in OMFS who are not registered with the GDC must be careful to know their legal limitations with respect to 'the practice of dentistry', which is defined and protected by law.

The practice of dentistry

Prior to 2005 it was acceptable for both registered dentists and doctors to practise dentistry. However, in 2005, following a judgement of the European Court of Justice,[1] the Dentists Act 1984 was amended, restricting the practice of dentistry to those with GDC registration.

Since the 2005 amendment, there has been some contention over what defines 'the practice of dentistry' with respect to OMFS, especially as the number of singly medically qualified doctors working in the specialty has steadily grown.

In 2008 a position statement on this issue was made by the GDC,[2] and subsequently reiterated by the British Association of Oral and Maxillofacial Surgeons (BAOMS).[3]

GDC statement

- 'The GDC considers that suitably qualified and registered healthcare professionals may take whatever action is necessary to deal with dental emergencies.'
- 'The GDC would expect any non-emergency dental treatment to be carried out by a GDC registrant.'
- 'Council would have no difficulty with suitably qualified and registered medical practitioners performing certain tasks, which would in a different context be restricted to GDC registrants (for example the extraction of teeth) if they are an essential part of a necessary medical or surgical procedure and are performed in that context.'
- 'This applies equally to oral and maxillofacial trainees and specialists.'

BAOMS statement

- 'Medical (non-GDC) registrants should be entitled to practice the full scope of OMFS, including the surgical removal of teeth and dental extractions, provided:
  - it is undertaken under the auspices of a hospital department of OMFS

---

1 Vogel, case c-35/02.
2 http://www.gdc-uk.org/NR/rdonlyres/563578AC-10D2-4A8B-A3FF-6B029F5E772E/76102/Practiceofdentristrystatement.doc.
3 http://www.baoms.org.uk/downloaddoc.asp?id=212.

- it is performed under appropriate supervision of and delegation from a consultant OMF surgeon
- the practitioner only undertakes treatments where they are competent to do so'.
- *"Council would not support a non-GDC registrant undertaking dental extractions or other dental procedures as an independent High Street practitioner"*.

Duties of an OMFS doctor

- OMFS is a very diverse specialty.
- In most OMFS units you will work with all age groups in all the main clinical areas.
- You will use a mixture of general medical knowledge and surgical skills, as well as a fair amount of dental knowledge and skills.
- You will also manage a diverse range of diseases from congenital oral anomalies in neonates to advanced disseminated cancer. You may be called upon to be an oral physician advising pediatricians on geographic tongue and following this find yourself in the A&E reducing a dislocated mandible or repairing a complex facial laceration.
- You should equip yourself with a good pen torch and some tongue spatulas. A miniature Snellen chart may also be useful.
- You will be expected to acquire some skills quite quickly and we advise you to read this book at least once before you start your new job and use it to direct your learning of new skills.
- Many OMFS units have junior doctors from a mixture of backgrounds. Junior doctors working in the department may or may not be considering a career in OMFS. There may even be some doubly qualified doctors awaiting a specialist training post.
- You will find it advantageous to work as a team—the singly qualified doctor's medical knowledge will help the singly qualified dentist and their dental knowledge will help the doctor.

The future of OMFS

- OMFS has changed hugely in the last 10 years and has become the dominant specialty in head and neck cancer and in orthognathic, craniofacial, and oral surgery.
- However, at the time of writing most juniors in OMFS units are singly qualified dentists and this is the most likely and important change in the future for the specialty.
- Dental deaneries are shaping the training they demand of their graduates and the specialty itself is questioning the safety of this situation.
- The change has been slow but is inevitable; units will employ more medically qualified doctors to work in their departments. This will have some impact on the type of work juniors do unsupervised, but in reality the days of leaving an OMFS senior house officer to' just get on with' a list of dental extractions is over.
- In the past most OMFS consultants took dentistry as their first degree and had a fair amount of oral surgery experience before furthering their OMFS skills. However, in recent years an increasing number of medically qualified doctors are embarking on dentistry as a second degree. Perhaps this book will encourage this—we sincerely hope so!
- No one knows how this trend will change the specialty, if at all, but the doctors choosing to take dentistry as a second degree seem to be some of the most highly motivated and talented trainees. This can only be good for the specialty and encourage its future evolution.
- The future of OMFS as a challenging and rewarding specialty is assured, and the changes highlighted above will further this.

Career pathways in OMFS

- The requirements for a specialist training post include dental and medical degrees. A minimum of 6 months training in OMFS is essential.
- Those who have a dental degree can often obtain a medical degree on a shortened course, and similarly some dental schools are now offering shortened courses for doctors.
- Dental graduates who wish to work in the NHS must have a provider number which is given on completion of a vocational training post in the UK. This is not a requirement for those who wish to train in OMFS. However, those who are about to embark on a medical degree as a second degree may find it easier to find work if they have an NHS provider number.
- Some experience in other head and neck specialties, such as ear, nose, and throat (ENT), plastic surgery, neurosurgery, and ophthalmology, may be advantageous.
- Applicants for specialist training posts in OMFS will have spent longer in undergraduate training than other specialties, and it is usually expected that they will have maximized the benefit of this extra time and have a CV to reflect this.
- Most OMFS surgeons are quite enthusiastic about their specialty and tend to be supportive of trainees. If you are considering a career in OMFS, it is a good idea to approach a consultant in OMFS and get some advice early.
- The BAOMS has trainee groups who can help you make the right career choice and we recommend you contact them through the BAOMS website (www.baoms.org.uk).

Basic knowledge

Anatomy of the teeth

Anatomy of a tooth

A tooth is made up of a crown, a neck, and root(s). Each tooth has an individual nerve supply, arterial supply, and venous drainage, all of which make up the pulp of the tooth which lies within the root canals and central pulpal cavity. Surrounding the pulp is organic dentine, which is tubular and porous in its structure. The crown of the tooth has an outer coating of enamel, which is ~2mm thick. This is a very hard inorganic layer with the purpose of biting through or chewing food. The roots have a thinner coating of cementum, and are 'suspended' in the supporting alveolar bone by the periodontal ligament (PDL). The PDL has its own blood supply, and provides the proprioceptive sensory feedback to the brain, localizing the position of each individual tooth when the supporting jaw bites on something or if the tooth is percussed.

Tooth surface terminology

- *Mesial*—closer to midline
- *Distal*—further away from midline
- *Buccal*—facing the cheeks
- *Labial*—facing the lips
- *Palatal*—facing the palate (upper teeth only)
- *Lingual*—facing the tongue (lower teeth only)
- *Occlusal*—the biting surface of a premolar/molar tooth
- *Incisal*—the biting edge of an incisor or canine tooth

Deciduous teeth (primary teeth)

There are 20 deciduous teeth, with the first erupting at 6–8 months and the last by 20–24 months.

Permanent teeth (secondary teeth)

There are usually 32 permanent teeth, although this can vary due to extractions, trauma, impacted teeth, or supernumary teeth. The first molars erupt at age 6; the third molars are the last to erupt at age 17–21.

Charting teeth

When documenting or charting teeth, the Zsigmondy–Palmer, chevron, or set-square system is used which places the teeth in a grid (as seen from the front of the mouth).

- Permanent teeth:

8 7 6 5 4 3 2 1	1 2 3 4 5 6 7 8
8 7 6 5 4 3 2 1	1 2 3 4 5 6 7 8

- Deciduous teeth:

e d c b a	a b c d e
e d c b a	a b c d e

The quadrants can also be numbered: upper right is 1, upper left is 2, lower left is 3, and lower right is 4. For example, if you were annotating an upper-right lateral incisor, it would be (12) A lower-left canine would be (33).

General rules of thumb

Dental undergraduates spend a long and unhappy time learning the various tooth morphologies, as each tooth is different and there may be variations. In OMFS, it is important to appreciate the general rules of thumb in this regard, which will help guide extractions or re-implantations.

Upper teeth roots

- 1s, 2s, and 3s have conical roots.
- 4s and 5s have either two fine roots or a flattened root.
- 6s and 7s have three large, often splayed, roots. The palatal root is often longer than than the two (mesial and distal) buccal roots.

Lower teeth roots

- 1s, 2s, and 3s often have flattened or oval-shaped roots.
- 4s and 5s have mostly single conical roots, but occasionally have two roots.
- 6s and 7s have two roots (mesial and buccal).

❶ Non-dentally qualified OMFS doctors may have to re-implant a tooth in A&E as part of emergency treatment (📖 see p. 199). If you are going to re-implant a tooth, ensure that it is the right way round! The best way to ensure this is to look at the crown to identify the buccal/labial surface and the palatal/lingual surface. Anteror teeth have flat labial surfaces facing the lips, and concave palatal/lingual surfaces facing the palate or tongue. Posterior teeth generally have taller flatter buccal surfaces facing the cheeks, and lower more bulbous surfaces facing the tongue or palate.

Anatomy of the oral cavity

- It is worth knowing oral anatomy in detail (Fig. 2.1) as it features strongly in OMFS. Dental graduates will have an advantage here, but many medical anatomy courses will have only glossed over it.
- The oral cavity is split anatomically into two parts. The **vestibule** is the space between the lip/cheeks and the teeth/gingivae. The **mouth proper** is the space within the dental arches, housed superiorly by the palate and inferiorly by the tongue and floor of mouth.
- Posteriorly, the oral cavity communicates with the oropharynx.

Gingivae

The gums provide a soft tissue seal around the teeth. They consist of thicker attached keratinized gingivae, which include the embrasure spaces between the teeth as interdental papillae. The attached gingivae extend into the vestibule to become loose alveolar non-keratinized mucosa at the mucogingival junction, often clearly seen as a darker red line. These anatomical differences in tissue laxity must be borne in mind when suturing the gingivae as otherwise they are easily torn.

Teeth

(📖 See Anatomy of the teeth, p. 10)

Palate

The palate forms the roof of the mouth and the floor of the nose. It is split into the anterior hard palate and the posterior soft palate.

Hard palate

This is the bony anterior two-thirds of the palate, formed by the palatine processes of the maxillae and the horizontal processes of the palatine bones. The nasopalatine nerve and sphenopalatine artery exit anteriorly through the incisive canal, and the greater palatine vessels and nerve exit posteriorly through the greater palatine foramina before running anteriorly beneath the palatal mucosa. The lesser palatine nerve and vessels also exit from this foramen, but travel posteriorly into the soft palate.

Soft palate

This is the fibromuscular posterior third of the palate, extending posteroinferiorly from the edge of the hard palate to form the uvula. This protects food from going up the back of the nose on swallowing. Laterally, two arches of mucosa in continuation from the soft palate form the tonsillar fossae—the palatoglossal arch anteriorly and the palatopharyngeal arch posteriorly. The palatine tonsils lie in these fossae.

Tongue (Fig. 2.2)

The tongue is a muscular organ involved in mastication, taste, swallowing, (deglutition), speech (articulation) and oral cleansing. It is composed of muscles covered with mucous membrane. The tongue has a dorsal and ventral surface.he dorsal surface of which is roughened due to the presence of lingual papillae.

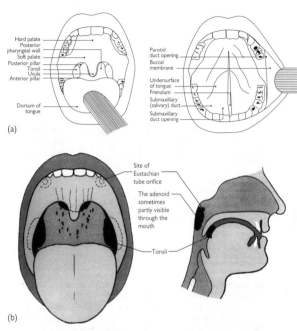

Fig. 2.1 (a) Mouth and throat structures. Reproduced from Corbridge R, Steventon N, *Oxford Handbook of ENT and Head and Neck Surgery*, p.187 (Oxford: 2010). With permission from Oxford University Press. (b) Oral cavity AP and oropharynx/nasopharynx lateral. Reproduced from Corbridge R, Steventon N *Oxford Handbook of ENT and Head and Neck Surgery*, p.185 (Oxford: 2010). With permission from Oxford University Press.

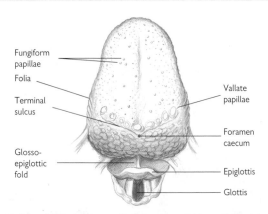

Fig. 2.2 External view of the tongue. Reproduced from Mackinnon P, Morris J, *Oxford Textbook of Functional Anatomy* Vol. 3, p.78 (Oxford: 2005). With permission from Oxford University Press.

The blood supply to the tongue is via the lingual artery, which arises from the external carotid artery and enters the tongue deep to the hypo-glossus muscle. Venous drainage is via the dorsal and deep lingual veins terminating in the internal jugular vein. The sensory nerve supply to ANTERIOR 2/3 of the tongue is the lingual nerve branch of CN V3, and taste is the chorda tympani branch of CN VII. The POSTERIOR 1/3 of the tongue is supplied by glossopharyngeal nerve (CN IX) for sensation and taste. Motor nerve supply is the hypoglossal nerve (CN XII) to all muscles except palatoglossus which is innervated by the vagus nerve (CN X).

Floor of the mouth

In the centre line is the fibrous lingual frenum with the two submandibular duct (**Wharton's duct**) openings at its base—the sublingual caruncle. The sublingual glands sit beneath the mucosa and create the sublingual ridges. The multiple **ducts of Rivinus** drain saliva produced by the sublingual gland into the floor of mouth along the sublingual ridges. A further single sublingual duct, the **duct of Bartholin**, also drains bilaterally at the sublingual caruncle. Lingual veins draining the tongue will be obvious to see, and the lingual nerve runs just mesial to the sublingual gland.

❶The floor of mouth tissues are loose and can swell quickly with cellulitis or oedema. This pushes the tongue upwards and backwards, and can obstruct the airway.

Retromolar trigone

This is the triangular area of mucosa behind the last standing lower molar, continuous with the maxillary tuberosity. The pterygomandibular raphe, just mesial to the trigone, connects the pterygoid process to the mylo-hyoid ridge of the mandible, and it is here that the buccinator muscle of the mouth and the superior constrictor muscle of the oropharynx attach. Therefore the retromolar trigone can be seen as a crossroads between the oral cavity, oropharynx, nasopharynx, buccinator space, and parapharyngeal space.

Anatomy of the facial skeleton

- The facial bones and cranium make up the skull (Fig. 2.3). The cranium encloses the brain, whilst the facial skeleton contains the eyes, nose, and mouth.
- The facial skeleton acts as a 'crumple zone', preferentially fracturing to absorb force directed at these structures during trauma.

Frontal bone

This is the skeleton of the forehead. It articulates inferiorly with the nasal bones at the nasion and the zygomas at the zygomatico-frontal suture. It also forms the roof of the orbit and superior orbital rim and contributes partly to the medial orbital wall. Within the frontal bone just above the nasion there are frontal air sinuses, which can crumple and fracture with trauma.

The orbits

The orbit is a pyramidal or cone-shaped cavity, with its base anterior and the apex posterior. The orbits protect the globe of the eye, the associated muscles, nerves, vessels, and the lacrimal apparatus. The orbit has four walls and an apex, made up of the following facial bones.

- Superior wall (thick)—frontal, lesser wing of sphenoid (near apex).
- Medial wall (thin)—ethmoid, frontal, lacrimal, lesser wing of sphenoid.
- Inferior wall (thin)—maxilla, zygomatic, palatine.
- Lateral wall (thick)—frontal process of zygomatic, greater wing of sphenoid.
- Apex—optic canal through lesser wing of sphenoid.

The naso-ethmoidal complex

The bony part of the nose consisting of:

- nasal bones
- frontal processes of maxillae
- nasal part of the frontal bone
- perpendicular plate of the ethmoid
- inferior conchae and vomer.

The shape of the external nose is governed by differences in the nasal cartilages. It is divided into two chambers by the partly bony and cartilaginous nasal septum, the main components of which are:

- perpendicular plate of ethmoid—superior (this descends from the cribiform plate of the ethmoid which separates the nasal cavity from the anterior cranial fossa; a broken nose or naso-ethmoidal complex can cause a dural tear and a CSF leak or can transmit infection from the nose into the brain meninges)
- vomer—posteroinferior
- septal cartilage—anterior.

Within the lateral mass of the ethmoidal bone are **ethmoid cells** which make up the ethmoid sinuses. If drainage is blocked, infection can pass from these cells through the fragile medial wall of the orbit and can cause (post-septal) periorbital cellulitis which, if not treated, can cause blindness.

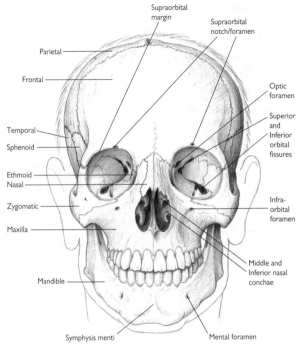

Fig. 2.3 The facial bones. Reproduced from Mackinnon P, Morris J, *Oxford Textbook of Functional Anatomy* Vol. 3, p.46 (Oxford: 2005). With permission from Oxford University Press.

The zygomatic complex

The zygomatic or malar bone forms the prominence of the cheek and also the lateral and partly inferior wall of the orbit. These bilateral bones have a central body with three processes—the frontal process, the temporal process and the maxillary process.

The maxilla

The upper jaw is formed by the fused maxillae. Their alveolar prominences support the maxillary teeth. The fused maxillae form a pyramidal shape, articulating bilaterally with the zygomatic bones and superiorly with the frontal bone and nasal bones. The maxilla also contributes to the floor of the orbits.

The mandible

The mandible forms the lower jaw and contributes to the temporomandibular joint. Its alveolar processes house the mandibular teeth. The mandible is a squared-off U-shape and so often fractures in more than one place. Figure 2.4 shows the various regions of the lower jaw, which are important when describing fractures (📖 see p. 66). The inferior alveolar branch of the trigeminal nerve runs through the mandible, exiting anteriorly through the mental foramina which are located between the roots of the lower premolar teeth bilaterally (Fig. 2.5). The condylar head of the mandible articulates within the glenoid fossa of the temporal bone, separated by an articular disc and controlled by ligaments and the muscles of mastication (📖 see Fig 2.8, p. 28).

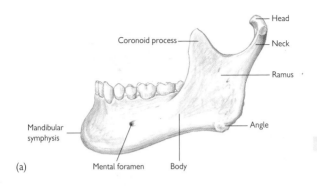

(a)

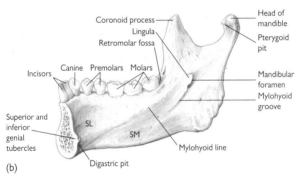

(b)

Fig. 2.4 Regions of the mandible: (a) lateral aspect; (b) medial aspect. SM, submandibular salivary gland; SL, sublingual salivary gland. Reproduced from Mackinnon P, Morris J, *Oxford Textbook of Functional Anatomy* Vol. 3, p.80 (Oxford: 2005). With permission from Oxford University Press.

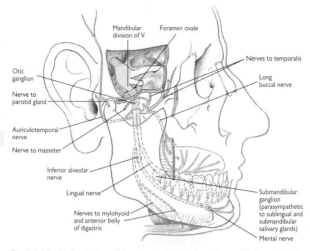

Fig. 2.5 Mandibular division of the trigeminal nerve (cranial nerve V). Reproduced from Mackinnon P, Morris J, *Oxford Textbook of Functional Anatomy* Vol. 3, p.78 (Oxford: 2005). With permission from Oxford University Press.

Dental occlusion

- Much of OMFS work involves dental occlusion, in particular facial hard tissue trauma, cancer resection/reconstruction, and orthognathic surgery.

Definitions

- **Occlusion**: in simple terms, means the contact between teeth.
- **Malocclusion**: a misalignment of the teeth and jaws: a 'bad bite'.
- **Centric occlusion**: the occlusion made when the jaw is closed and the teeth meet together in maximum interdigitation. Ask the patient to bite down on their back teeth and view from each side with a pen torch.
- **Ideal occlusion**: anatomically perfect occlusion based on the classifications listed below and various other factors. Ideal occlusion is rare.
- **Lateral excursions**: lateral movements of the mandible to each side.
- **Anterior open bite**: a space exists between the upper and lower incisors when viewed from the front, and the teeth are otherwise in occlusion. Lateral open bite is a space existing on one side.
- **Crossbite**: teeth are displaced either buccally or lingually. Can be anterior/posterior and unilateral/bilateral.
- **Overbite**: the extent of overlap of the upper central incisors over the lower central incisors when viewed from the front.
- **Overjet**: the extent of the protrusion of the upper teeth ahead of the lower teeth when viewed from the side. Can be termed a 'reverse overjet' if the lower teeth are protruding ahead of the upper teeth.
- **Occlusal vertical dimension (OVD)**: the height of the two jaws, or lower face height.
- **Orthodontics**: a dental specialty concerned with growth of the face, development of the teeth, and prevention/treatment of occlusal problems.
- **Orthognathic surgery**: surgery to correct abnormalites in facial skeleton growth, or structure causing severe malocclusions. Can have functional and/or aesthetic indications.

Classifications of occlusion

British Standards Institute (BSI) classification (Fig. 2.6)

Based on the incisor relationship.

- *Class I (ideal)*: the incisal edge of the lower incisor contacts or lies below the cingulum of the upper central incisor (Fig. 2.6(a)).
  (A cingulum is a convexity found on the lingual surface of anterior teeth. It is identifiable as an inverted V-shaped ridge.)
- *Class II*: the incisal edge of the lower incisor lies posterior to the cingulum of the upper incisor. There are two types.
  - *Division I*: the upper incisors are proclined or of an average inclination and there is an increased overjet (Fig. 2.6(b)).
  - *Division II*: the upper central incisors are retroclined (Fig. 2.6(c)).
- *Class III*: the incisal edges of the lower incisor lie anterior to the cingulum plateau of the upper incisors (Fig. 2.6(d)).

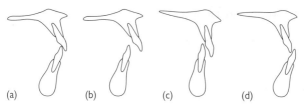

Fig. 2.6 BSI classification. Reproduced from Mitchell L, Mitchell D, *Oxford Handbook of Clinical Dentistry* (5th edn), p.125 (Oxford: 2009). With permission from Oxford University Press.

Occlusion can also be classified based on the relationship between upper and lower canine teeth and molar teeth.

Skeletal factors
As the teeth are set in the jaws, the relationship of the jaws to one another has an influence on the dental arches.

The antero-posterior skeletal pattern
- *Skeletal I*: the jaws are in their ideal antero-posterior relationship in occlusion
- *Skeletal II*: the lower jaw in occlusion is positioned more posteriorly
- *Skeletal III*: the lower jaw in occlusion is positioned more anteriorly.

Factors causing malocclusion

Genetic factors
- Skeletal factors
- Tooth size and number

Metabolic factors
For example, a pituitary adenoma secreting growth hormone resulting in progressive malocclusion usually presenting in middle to late age.

Environmental factors
- Soft tissue factors: lips, cheeks, and tongue can either move or stabilize teeth over time.
- Habits: thumb/finger sucking, pen biting. etc.
- Trauma: fractured mandible or midface, traumatized dentition.
- Temporomandibular joint (TMJ) dislocation.

Local factors
- Variation in number of teeth
- Spaced teeth

Problems caused by malocclusion

Teeth
Teeth can break or wear, crowns or fillings can come loose, teeth can ache or move.

Soft tissue
Gums can recede.

Temporomandibular joint
Clicking, grinding, locking, pain, trismus, headache, tinnitus, muscle fatigue and spasms, headache, sinus/eye pain, neck/back pain.

Functional
Difficult biting or chewing.

Patient aesthetic concerns
Altered appearance from the norm.

Anatomy of the oral and facial muscles, nerves, and glands

Muscles
- Facial muscles (Fig. 2.7)
- Muscles of mastication (Fig. 2.8)

Nerves

Lingual nerve
Branch of trigeminal (CN V); passes medial to the mandible, close to the posterior molar teeth into the posterolateral tongue where it supplies sensation to the anterior two-thirds of the tongue. It also lies in close apposition to the deep lobe of the submandibular gland. It crosses the submandibular duct.

Inferior alveolar nerve (or inferior dental nerve (IDN))
Branch of trigeminal (CN V); enters the mandible posteriorly at the lingua to pass through the body of the mandible anteriorly where it then exits via the mental foramen as the **mental nerve** to supply sensation to the lower lip and chin. It passes close to the apices of the posterior molar teeth and so can be damaged during dento-alveolar surgery.

Facial nerve
The facial nerve (CN VII) exits the skull base through the stylomastoid foramen. As it passes through the parotid gland, it splits into five main divisions: temporal, zygomatic, buccal, marginal mandibular, and cervical (Fig. 2.9). These branches supply facial movements—eyebrow raise/frown, eye squint, cheeks, mouth.

The marginal mandibular branch of CN VII runs just deep to the platysma and loops below the level of the mandible, which is why a skin excision (e.g. during submandibular gland excision or extra-oral drainage of a dentofacial abscess) should be made at least two finger breadths inferior to the mandible to avoid iatrogenic damage to this nerve. The facial nerve is also sensory to the upper pole of the tonsil and part of the external auditory meatus.

Glands

Parotid gland
This pyramid-shaped gland lies behind the angle of the mandible and in front of the ear, covered by a thick parotid fascia. Serous saliva produced by the gland is expressed into the mouth via **Stenson's duct** at the parotid papilla inside the cheek opposite the upper second molar tooth. The gland contains the external carotid artery, which divides into the maxillary and superficial temporal branches within the gland (deep to the facial nerve). Facial nerve division within the gland is described above.
- Innervation: glossopharyngeal nerve (CN IX) via auriculotemporal nerve—parasympathetic stimulation.
- Blood supply: transverse facial artery.

SUPERFICIAL MUSCLES

DEEPER MUSCLES

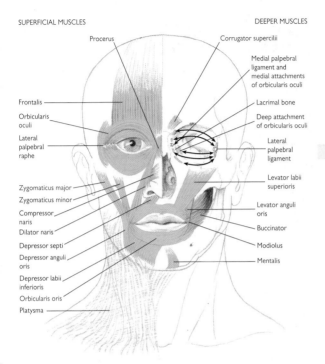

Fig. 2.7 Facial muscles. Reproduced from Mackinnon P, Morris J, *Oxford Textbook of Functional Anatomy* Vol. 3, p.67 (Oxford: 2005). With permission from Oxford University Press.

Submandibular gland

This bi-lobed gland lies beneath the mandible just anterior to its angle. The superficial and deep lobes are separated by the posterior free edge of the mylohyoid. The gland produces a mixed serous/mucinous saliva, and this is expressed into the mouth via **Wharton's duct** which runs from the deep lobe of the gland along the floor of the mouth to the papillae located either side of the tongue frenum.

- Innervation: via submandibular ganglion.
- Blood supply: facial artery.

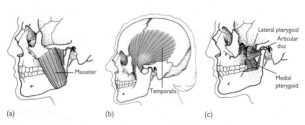

Fig. 2.8 Muscles of mastication: (a) masseter; (b) temporalis; (c) pterygoid muscles (coronoid process of mandible removed). Reproduced from Mackinnon P, Morris J, *Oxford Textbook of Functional Anatomy* Vol. 3, p.83 (Oxford: 2005). With permission from Oxford University Press.

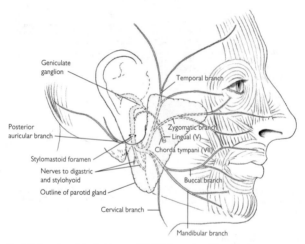

Fig. 2.9 Branches of the facial nerve (CN VII). Reproduced from Mackinnon P, Morris J, *Oxford Textbook of Functional Anatomy* Vol. 3, p.80 (Oxford: 2005). With permission from Oxford University Press.

Anatomy of the neck

Surface anatomy

The sternocleidomastoid muscle (SCM) is the key anatomical landmark in the neck, splitting it diagonally into anterior and posterior triangles, with the trapezius muscles making up the posterior aspect of the neck. Further triangle subdivisions are described (Fig. 2.10).

Within the triangles of the neck, various superficial structures can be seen or palpated (Fig. 2.11). It is worth knowing the neck landmarks for emergency procedures, such as a needle or surgical cricothyroidectomy, and for other elective operations, such as tracheostomy, thyroidectomy and submandibular gland excision, which are described in the emergency and operative chapters of this book.

Fascial layers

Superficial cervical fascia

This is a subcutaneous connective tissue layer containing the platysma, cutaneous nerves, blood vessels, and lymphatics.

Deep cervical fascia

- The **investing fascia** surrounds all the structures in the neck.
- The **pre-vertebral fascia** divides the neck into anterior and posterior compartments. The posterior compartment contains the vertebral column and its associated muscles. Deep to this fascia is the phrenic nerve (C3,4,5) and brachial plexus.
- The anterior compartment contains further deep fascial envelopes:
  - the **pre-tracheal fascia** encloses the thyroid, trachea, pharynx, and oesophagus
  - the **carotid sheath** encases the common and internal carotid arteries, the internal jugular vein, the vagus nerve (CN X), the deep cervical lymph nodes, the carotid sinus nerve, and sympathetic fibres.

The deep fascial layers form natural cleavage planes through which tissues may be separated during surgery. they limit spread of abscesses resulting from infections, and allow structures to move and slide over each other when twisting the neck or swallowing. It is important to have a good working knowledge of the fascial spaces of the neck for better understanding of the spread of dentofacial infections (Fig. 2.11).

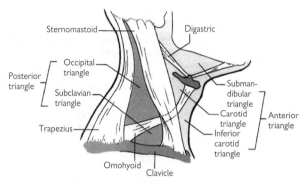

Fig. 2.10 Triangles of the neck. Reproduced from Corbridge R, Steventon N, *Oxford Handbook of ENT and Head and Neck Surgery*, p.262 (Oxford: 2010). With permission from Oxford University Press.

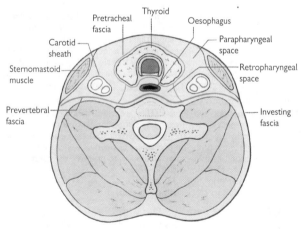

Fig. 2.11 Fascial layers and spaces of the neck. Reproduced from Corbridge R, Steventon N, *Oxford Handbook of ENT and Head and Neck Surgery*, p.263 (Oxford: 2010). With permission from Oxford University Press.

Muscles

Platysma

Originates from fascia of pectoralis major/deltoid and inserts into tip of chin and mandible. Fibres also blend with those of muscles of lower face. Innervation: cervical branch of VII (on its deep surface). Actions: draws corners of mouth down and depresses mandible. Soft tissue injuries that penetrate this muscle layer must be explored in theatre.

Sternocleidomastoid

Rotates head to opposite side. Originates from mastoid process of temporal bone, inserts into manubrium and clavicle. Innervation: spinal root of accessory nerve (CN XI) and C2/3.

Suprahyoid and infrahyoid (strap) muscles

See Figure 2.12.

Glands

Thyroid gland

This gland saddles the larynx and the trachea and is surrounded by the pretracheal fascia. It consists of two lobes joined in the midline by the isthmus. It is a highly vascular gland supplied by the superior and inferior thyroid arteries and occasionally a third inominate or 'thyroid ima' artery (~1%) which can run directly off the arch of aorta supplying the gland from below. This can present a problem during tracheostomy.

The paired recurrent laryngeal nerves are located just posterior to the thyroid gland and can be damaged by thyroid surgery or invaded by thyroid malignancy, causing a weak breathy voice. Innervation is via the cervical sympathetic ganglia.

Parathyroid glands

These vary in position and number. They are usually found embedded on the posterior aspect of the thyroid lobes. If performing a total thyroidectomy, the parathyroid glands (not always possible to preserve all four) must be located and left with their blood supply as removal will cause hypocalcaemia. A subtotal thyroidectomy would aim to preserve the parathyroid glands by leaving a posterior cuff of thyroid tissue.

- Blood supply: inferior thyroid arteries.
- Innervation: via cervical sympathetic ganglia.

Lymphatics of the neck

- Superfical cervical lymph nodes are located along the external and internal jugular veins. They drain into the deep cervical nodes.
- Deep cervical lymph nodes form a chain along the internal jugular vein, mostly under cover of the SCM.
- Other deep lymph node groups include the pre-laryngeal, pre-tracheal, para-tracheal, and retro-pharyngeal lymph nodes.

The lymph nodes of the neck are often classified according to their anatomical level within the neck (Fig. 2.13).

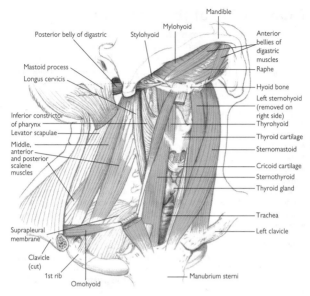

Fig. 2.12 Suprahyoid and infrahyoid muscles. Reproduced from Mackinnon P, Morris J, *Oxford Textbook of Functional Anatomy* Vol. 3, p.60 (Oxford: 2005). With permission from Oxford University Press.

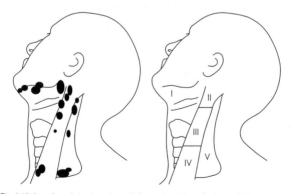

Fig. 2.13 Lymph node levels in the neck. Reproduced from Corbridge R, Steventon N, *Oxford Handbook of ENT and Head and Neck Surgery*, p.263 (Oxford: 2010). With permission from Oxford University Press.

Examination of the oral cavity

The oral cavity extends from the vermilion border of the lips to the anterior pillar of fauces where it becomes the oropharynx. Although the tonsils are in the oropharynx, it is good practice to examine them also.

❶Examination of the neck is mandatory in conjunction with the oral cavity. If you examine the neck first, you won't forget to do so afterwards. Record both positive and negative findings. (📖 see p. 37)

The keys to good oral examination are:
• be systematic
• wear gloves
• get a good light source
• have gauze and suction available
• support the head
• extend the neck
• be calm and gentle, and tell the patient what you are about to do
• enquire if the tissues are painful before starting to examine
• use tongue spatulas or dental mirrors for retraction
• be aware of the gag reflex.

Examination
• Look first using **two** mirrors or spatulas to retract the cheeks or lips as you will see more if you keep your hands out of the way.
• Examine the lips, buccal mucosa, hard and soft palate, gingivae, teeth, retromolar trigone, tonsils, and dorsal tongue.
• Hold the tongue-end with gauze and, with the patient's help, move it to one side and examine the floor of the mouth and the ventral tongue.
• Mucosal lesions may be better examined after drying with gauze.
• Palpate any lesions you find. Texture is important (the hard 'grittiness' of malignancy is a valuable sign).
• Palpate the lips, cheeks, and tongue, especially the base of tongue.
• The floor of the mouth and the submandibular gland are best palpated bimanually (gloved finger of one hand inside the mouth and other hand pressing up from the neck).
• Milk saliva from the parotid and submandibular glands, looking for volume, consistency, and pus or debris.
• Examine cranial nerves, especially facial, trigeminal, hypoglossal and palato-pharyngeal plexus.

Additional tests

Vitality testing of teeth
Using an electric pulp tester or just ethyl chloride sprayed onto a cotton wool pledget placed onto the tooth surface will give you an indication of whether the pulp is alive or dead (not always reliable).

Percussion of teeth

This will be painful if there is periapical or lateral inflammation of the periodontal ligament, such as acute apical periodontitis secondary to pulpal infection. NB: the periodontal ligament must be inflamed for the tooth to be tender on percussion. If infection is confined to the pulp only (i.e pulpitis), percussion may not evoke a positive response.

Use of probes

Probes can be used to investigate periodontal pockets as well as periodontal sinuses. Occasionally a gutta percha point carefully inserted into a sinus followed by a periapical radiograph will show the source of the sinus. This technique can also be useful in confirming a small oro-antral fistula.

Small lacrimal probes can also be used to dilate salivary ducts and strictures.

Radiographs

Useful for dental disease, bone lesions, soft tissue foreign bodies, and salivary calculi. Many departments have equipment in the clinic. (📖 see Chapter 3, Radiology)

Nasendoscopy

Unidentified neck lumps and head and neck cancer referrals necessitate a nasendoscopy. (📖 see p. 206)

Examination of the face and neck

- Be systematic. Try to adopt a structured approach so that pathology is not missed.
- As always, good light and access will help, and if there is a dental chair available, use it. You can then recline the patient and walk around the head-end, easily examining from different angles.
- Always note down examination findings in detail, as the clinical picture can often change with time.

The face

Soft tissues

A close inspection of the soft tissues is required first, bearing in mind that signs of trauma and pathology can often be missed within the patient's hair and around the ears. Examine for asymmetry, masses, scars, or deformity. Having established if the patient is tender anywhere, gently palpate the soft tissues, gently comparing each side of the midline. If a swelling or mass is present, note the following.

- ❶ Site, size, shape, surface, colour, temperature, consistency, fluctuance, fixity, and pulsatility, and whether there are other associated signs such as a punctum or local lymphadenopathy.
- ❶ With any abnormality on the skin surface, immediately think about associated deeper anatomy such as bones, muscles, nerves, blood vessels, lymphatics, and underlying glands or ducts.

Hard tissues

The facial skeleton should be examined systematically, bearing in mind that there may be signs pointing to fractures in the overlying soft tissues, such as contusion, bruising, haematoma, swelling, laceration, and crepitus.

When palpating the facial bones, compare both sides of the face, feeling for step deformities, depressions, movement, or sharp bone fracture ends.

Eyes

- Examine the eyes for abnormalities of the sclera, iris, and pupil.
- A subconjunctival haemorrhage is an important sign to note, particularly if there is no posterior limit to the haemorrhage, as it may mean there is an orbital wall fracture.
- Pupillary reflexes, eye movements, and fundoscopy should be examined as part of the cranial nerve examination.
- Visual acuity should always be recorded for any trauma involving the eye or surrounding facial tissues.
- Examine the conjunctivae and eyelids. Look for proptosis, lid retraction, or ptosis.
- Check intercanthal distance and interpupillary distance.

Nose

- Look externally for deformity, asymmetry, or skin lesions.
- Look internally for septal deviation or haematoma. Assess air entry bilaterally. Check for signs of bleeding or discharge.

Ears
- Look for deformity, haematoma, or skin lesions.
- Use an auroscope to look into the ear, check that the auditory canal is patent and that the tympanic membrane is intact.
- Check for signs of bleeding or discharge.

The neck

Examination steps
- Inspect from the front and the side before standing behind the patient to palpate the neck. Ask the patient to swallow (thyroid mass).
- Use two hands to palpate left and right sides simultaneously for comparison.
- Move methodically to palpate all lymphatic chains, starting under the chin and moving backward to palpate the submandibular region.
- The submandibular gland must be differentiated from submandibular nodes. The gland can often be appreciated better by placing a gloved finger in the floor of mouth so that it can be palpated bimanually.
- Continue to examine over the angle of mandible, the pre-auricular and parotid region, and the post-auricular region, and then move down the SCM muscle.
- Try to displace the muscle gently so that deeper nodes are not missed.
- Don't forget the supraclavicular areas, before carefully examining the midline and thyroid gland.
- Finish by examining the posterior triangle of the neck.
- (☐ see Triangles of the neck, Fig 2.10, p.31).

Thyroid gland examination
Examination of the thyroid requires a specific approach in addition to the neck examination, and is an examiner's favourite.
- Look at the skin in general and hair quality, including the lateral third of the eyebrows, which can be lost in hypothyroidism.
- Look at the eyes for signs of exophthalmos or lid lag seen in hyper-thyroidism.
- Ask the patient to swallow, inspecting the neck from the front. A thyroid mass will rise during swallowing. Check for any scars of previous surgery.
- The gland should be palpated from behind, comparing the right and left lobes and the isthmus between them. A normal gland will most likely be impalpable.
- Distinguish any other midline neck swelling from what could be a thyroid isthmus swelling, e.g. a thyroglossal cyst will rise when a patient protrudes their tongue rather than on swallowing.
- Percussion may identify a goitre with retrosternal extension.
- Auscultate for bruits associated with vascular hyperactive thyroid glands.
- Other thyroid-specific examination points are to listen to the voice (a weak, hoarse, or breathy voice might indicate a recurrent laryngeal nerve palsy from invading malignancy or previous surgery) and examine the hands (sweaty palms or a resting tremor could indicate hyper-thyroidism).

Radiology

Guidelines for dental radiology

General points

- Although the radiation doses are generally quite low, the same rules apply as with other radiology and are controlled by IRMER (Ionizing Radiation (Medical Exposure) Regulations (2000)).
  - Does patient really need the radiograph?
  - Will it change your management?
  - Make sure you get the best investigation for the case. If in doubt talk to a radiologist
  - Ensure that the request form carries all information
  - Don't do it unless you or someone else has the ability to interpret the result
- The taking and interpretation of dental radiographs is part of the dental undergraduate curriculum. The same is not true of most doctors and you must not be tempted into taking dental radiographs unless you are trained to do so.
- Interpretation can be difficult. Get some help—your dental colleagues will be willing and able.
- Pregnant patients can have dental radiographs (the exposure of the fetus to radiation is virtually nil), but again only if the radiograph is necessary. Use a lead apron and if possible aim the beam away from the abdomen.
- One of the most common errors with dental radiographs is mislabelling or wrong-siding, so always double check that you have the correct radiograph and that it is the right way round before you act on it, especially for irreversible procedures such as dental extractions.
- Likewise, take pains to ensure that any hard-copy dental films you acquire are correctly labelled, sided, and filed.
- To avoid taking unnecessary radiographs the referring dentist may send you their films. These are useful, so always enquire if they are available and make efforts to obtain them. Likewise, make an effort to ensure that they are returned after you have finished with them—this is always appreciated by the referring practitioner.

Dental radiography

Dental radiographs
- As far as this book is concerned all dental radiographs involve a film (either an X-ray film or a digital X-ray plate) positioned intra-orally. They are used for examining the teeth or tissues immediately around the teeth.
- Other radiographs, such as dental panoramic tomograms (DPTs; also called OPGs), although used by dentists, are better for imaging the jaws and as such are considered later with other craniofacial radiography.

Periapical radiographs (Fig. 3.1)
- Dentists tend to use term 'PA' for periapical whilst most in radiology use PA to mean postero-anterior so don't be confused.
- Good periapical radiographs are difficult to take and few radiology departments outside dental schools will attempt them.
- For this reason many OMFS departments have their own intra-oral radiology equipment. Don't use it unless you are trained to do so.
- Periapicals can be uncomfortable, especially for lower posterior teeth, and it is rarely possible to obtain a view of lower wisdom teeth, so most surgeons rely on DPT for wisdom tooth assessment.
- Upper anterior periapical views are also difficult and a standard upper occlusal may be better.

Indications for periapical radiographs
- Apical pathology, loss of bone, cyst, etc.
- Assessment of periodontal ligament width (increased with inflammation).
- Looking at roots for fracture or resorption, or checking morphology prior to extraction.
- To see root canal and apex as part of endodontic treatment or to look for resorption or foreign body.
- May show unerupted teeth and can be used in parallax.
- Can be used in implantology to check position and integration.
- Will show loss of the dense white line around the tooth root which represents the compact bone (lamina dura). This will be lost if teeth are being moved by an orthodontist or if a tooth is ankylosed. Also lost in systemic diseases such as hyperparathyroidism.

Bitewing radiographs
- 'Bitewings' are the usual dental investigation for dental caries.
- They do not show the apex of tooth.
- They can also be used to assess the periodontal status and bone height.
- They are not much use for anything else and are rarely used in OMFS.

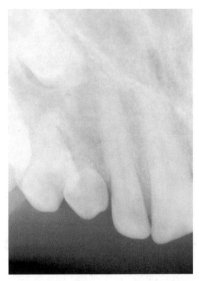

Fig. 3.1 Periapical showing upper right incisor region. Note the detail that this radiograph can give.

Occlusal radiographs (Fig. 3.2)

- Broadly divided into upper or lower occlusal.
- Lower occlusal are 'true' if the beam is at 90° to the film, and 'oblique left or right' and 'standard' if the beam is at 45° to the film.
- Upper occlusal can be 'left or right oblique', 'vertex' if the beam is parallel to the upper incisors and 'standard' if at 90° to the film.
- You probably do not need a vertex occlusal and a lot of radiation passes through the brain, so forget it! If you are considering it to look for unerupted upper canines, try the parallax technique.

Indication for occlusal radiographs

- Upper occlusal in combination with other radiographs such as DPT can be used in parallax.
- Upper standard occlusal is like having a periapical of the front four teeth and the indications are the same.
- It is also useful for assessing the nasopalatine canal or nasomaxillary cysts.
- Upper occlusal can be useful to show root fractures, which can be hard to see with periapical if the beam is at right angles to the fracture.
- Lower oblique can show a stone in the anterior part of the sub-mandibular duct.
- Lower occlusal can show fractures of the anterior mandible which sometimes do not show well on a PA of the mandible.

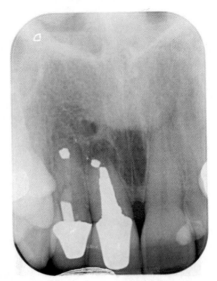

Fig. 3.2 This upper occlusal shows good detail of anterior teeth. Note the apical pathology on UR1. Both teeth have amalgam retrograde root fillings. The superimposed shadow is the nasal tip.

The parallax technique (Fig. 3.3)

- Used when planning removal of unerupted upper canines to show if tooth is lying on the palatal or buccal side of the jaw. This determines which side of the jaw the surgeon approaches, so is quite important.
- The principle is to take two radiographs of unerupted tooth from different angles in either the horizontal or vertical plane.
- Then compare the two films, thinking how the orientation of the beam of radiation has moved from one film to the other.
- If the unerupted tooth appears to have moved from one film to the other in same direction as the beam has moved from one film to the other, it is on palatal side ('your pal moves with you').
- Conversely if the tooth moves in the opposite direction, it is buccal. If it does not move, it is probably in line with the dental arch or else your radiographs have not been taken at sufficiently different angles to show an effect!
- The most common combination is a DPT and an upper occlusal. If the canine appears to be more vertically positioned compared with, say, the lateral incisor on the upper occlusal film than on the DPT, it is palatally positioned.
- There are other ways to tell. You can get a lateral view or a cone beam CT (CBCT) or you could rely on clinical signs see 'in clinics' impacted teeth and 'in theatre' impacted teeth.

OPG

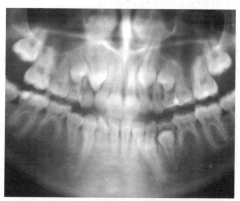

Upper occlusal

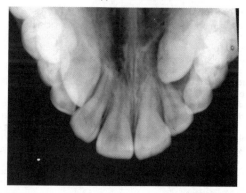

Fig. 3.3 OPG and upper occlusal views of impacted upper canines. Note that on going from OPG to upper occlusal the X-ray machine orientation moves from horizontal for the OPG to more vertical for the upper occlusal, so the position of the canine on the left moves nearer the apex of the lateral incisor, i.e. as the X-ray cone moves up so does the tooth. Therefore it is palatal (your pal moves with you). On the right there is no movement; it is in the line of the arch. These radiographs were kindly supplied by Mr Vicor Crow, Consultant Orthodontist at North West London Hospitals.

Panoramic radiography

The dental panoramic tomogram (Fig. 3.4)
- Otherwise known as DPT, OPG, or OPT.
- This is the most commonly used radiograph in OMFS.
- It is equivalent in terms of radiation exposure to about four periapical radiographs, and far lower than a chest X-ray.
- It involves the beam and the film rotating around the patient and imaging everything within the focal trough.
- It only shows the structures within the trough or focal section.
- The focal trough is horseshoe shaped.
- Ideally, the trough includes all the teeth, the whole of the mandible, and most of the maxilla.
- Structures outside the trough are blurred.
- The technique generates a lot of artefacts, especially from jewelry.
- Taking a DPT requires some degree of cooperation from the patient, and rarely gives worthwhile results with the inebriated, the severely physically or mentally disabled, or the very young.
- The anterior region is usually poorly defined in both jaws because of superimposition of the cervical vertebrae.

Indications for DPT
- General dental assessment (e.g. prior to head and neck radiotherapy).
- General periodontal assessment—will show bone loss.
- Bone pathology, cysts, fibro-osseous lesions, cancer, etc.
- Bone morphology, asymmetry, hyperplasia, etc.
- Fractures; in combination with another film such as PA jaws, will show most jaw fractures and anterior mandible fractures which are difficult to see because of the spine.
- Wisdom teeth—shows presence, orientation, and relationship to inferior alveolar canal to some extent. If in doubt, CBCT is better.
- Will show if maxillary sinus is clear but is not useful for assessing sinus pathology. It cannot rule out sinus cancer, for example, and may only show the root in the sinus if it is within the trough; if near midline, it may not show. Might show OAC.
- Can be used to assess articular surfaces of TMJ, although CT is better. MRI scan is used to assess for internal derangement of the joint in selected cases only!
- Commonly used in implantology, although the degree of magnification can be an issue. However, this can be overcome. For more accuracy CBCT is better.
- Occasionally used to show radio-opaque stones in the submandibular system.

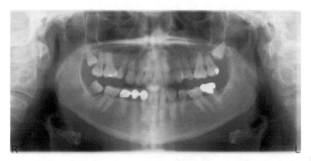

Fig. 3.4 A fairly typical DPT showing periodontal disease around the lower right last standing molar, impacted upper wisdom teeth, root fillings, bridgework, and restorations.

Facial and skull radiography

General points

- The main indications for craniofacial radiographs are fractures, benign and malignant tumours, developmental anomalies, and other rare conditions.
- Because these radiographs require a higher dose of radiation around the brain and eyes, it is particularly important that you order the most appropriate film for the condition you are managing. There are likely to be protocols for most things, and there are some films that departments will not take unless specifically requested by a consultant (e.g. submento-vertex view for assessing the zygomatic arch).
- For assessment of craniofacial fractures you need two radiographs at different angles, ideally at 90° to each other.
- We will outline most common uses of craniofacial radiographs below, but if in doubt ask before you order. You can't un-irradiate someone! Giving unnecessary radiation could also be regarded as assault, so be warned!

Occipitomental (OM) views (Fig. 3.5)

- Followed by angle of beam to the horizontal, which can be 0° or 30°.
- If someone says 'OM45' they are probably referring to 'OM0'. However, '45' the angle of the head to the vertical plate with the beam at 0°, which is confusing but is irrelevant for most of us as long as we get two OM views at different angles.
- OM0 shows the facial skeleton and maxillary sinus without the dense bones of base of skull getting in the way, and so is used for fractures of the midface, zygomas, and orbits (Fig. 3.4).
- OM30 is required in combination with OM0 to ensure that fractures have not been missed, so it has the same indication as OM0 but is also useful for showing the coronoid process of the mandible.

Postero-anterior (PA) view of the jaws

- Shows the posterior part of mandible, including condyles, and the complete lower border of mandible.
- Useful for lesions in the mandible ramus to assess buccal–lingual expansion (e.g. cysts, ameloblastomas, etc.).
- Useful in combination with DPT to show fractures of mandible, but again will not show the anterior mandible well.
- Can help assessment of jaw asymmetry such as hyperplasia.

Lateral cephalogram

- Otherwise known as 'lateral ceph'.
- This is a standardized and reproducible lateral view of the face and anterior skull—an earpiece localizes the skull in the same place.
- Used by orthodontists and orthognathic surgeons to assess the PA relationships of the jaws and teeth.
- Some people use it to assess position of impacted upper canines.
- It is not used for much else. The non-standardized equivalent is the lateral skull, which is not used for much except occasionally to show anterior skull fractures and maxillary posterior fracture–displacement.

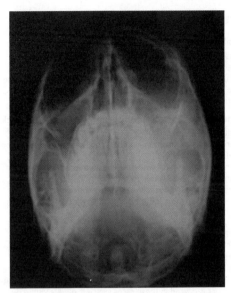

Fig. 3.5 OM view of fractured right zygomatic complex. Reproduced from Kerawala C, Newlands C, *Oxford Specialist Handbook of Oral and Maxillofacial Surgery*, p.47 (Oxford: 2010). With permission from Oxford University Press.

Lateral oblique view of mandible

- These are occasionally used to show the posterior mandible when the patient cannot have an DPT for whatever reason.
- If done well they are useful for fractures of the angle of mandible or assessment of wisdom teeth or other pathology in that region.

Other views

- Soft tissue views are occasionally used to assess foreign bodies in the lips or cheeks, although glass is not always visible (CBCT is better).
- There are other views of the craniofacial skeleton that are very occasionally used including reverse Townes (condyle), submentovertex (zygomatic arch), oblique PA jaws, etc.
- These are rarely useful and often radiology departments will not be happy doing them.
- If you are asked to arrange one of these unusual views, it is wise to know why beforehand, as radiology will want to know! Also, who will be able to interpret the resulting image?
- Most of these views have been superseded by CT or CBCT.

Skull radiographs are rarely useful in trauma cases and will not be discussed further here.

Ultrasonography

General points

- Because there is plenty of relatively superficial soft tissue in the head and neck; ultrasonography is generally very useful.
- It is only as good as the person performing and interpreting the images (at the same time), so it is hard to be dogmatic about its uses. Some departments get much more out of the service than others.

Main indications for ultrasonography in head and neck

- Neck lumps.
  - Can assess size, position, number, solid or cystic, shape, blood flow, and other features.
  - Can be used to guide fine-needle aspiration cytology (FNAC).
  - Can be used sequentially to monitor nodes on borderline between benign and suspicious features with inconclusive FNAC.
  - Used to distinguish solid, cystic, and single thyroid lumps from multiple lumps.
- Salivary gland disease.
  - Will show tumours within major salivary glands.
  - Will not show parotid tumours deep to the ramus mandible, MRI is better in these cases.
  - Will show salivary calculi in parotid and submandibular systems. May be difficult to see stones in submandibular duct (but often the duct is dilated in these cases which is readily visible on ultrasound (US)).
  - May show cysts of the major glands and can also be used for FNAC.
- Abscesses.
  - Can be used to see if there is a collection of pus within a swelling.
  - Can be used to assess extent of neck swelling, but in the face US may be hindered by bones shielding deep areas. Contrast-enhanced CT or MRI is better.
  - In reality, clinical assessment alone is often adequate and US may delay progress to theatre.
- Other uses.
  - Masseteric hypertrophy.
  - Vascular malformations.
  - Oral squamous cell carcinoma (SCC) thickness using intra-oral probe.
  - Duplex assessment of blood flow, looking for vessels in neck or potential free flap for reconstruction cases. For example, is there three-vessel run-off at the knee before we take the peroneal vessel out?
  - Lump over parotid—can be nice to be sure that the epidermoid cyst is actually that and not a parotid tumour. It happens!

CT and cone beam CT

General points

- CT and CBCT are great for visualizing the dental and bony structures of the head and neck and to a lesser extent the soft tissues. However, they involve more radiation than plain films and therefore their use must be justified.
- In emergency cases don't send the patient into a CT scanner if they have an impending airway crisis, uncontrolled bleeding, or other medical problem.
- The more you talk to the CT staff before scanning, the better the chance of getting what you want.
- Remember that not all the information from the scan will be available for you to see, so if you cannot see what you want, talk to the radiologist/radiographers in the CT suite and they may be able to make it available or reconfigure the images.
- For contrast-enhanced CT you need a recent renal function and a venflon—the radiologist will be your friend if one is already cited and viable!

CT and trauma

- In cases of severe craniofacial trauma most units have a low threshold of doing CT brain and/or cervical spine, so get involved quickly and arrange for the patient to have CT face done at same time. This saves them going back to scanner later. Your team will also be very pleased with you for that.
- For facial trauma you need fine slices and coronal reformatting. If your hospital gets a lot of facial trauma, the radiographer will know the sequences. But don't assume that they do—it might be their first day.
- 3D reconstruction is very helpful for complex craniofacial trauma— again, ask for it.
- Fractures of the orbit are very difficult to assess on plain films and most would advocate CT.
- Simple mandibular fractures rarely warrant CT, but it can be useful in comminuted fractures and/or complex condylar injuries.
- CT angiograms have a role in assessing and sometimes managing vascular injury in head and neck trauma (radiologists can embolize branches of the external carotid), so have that in the back of your mind when you talk to your registrar. However, don't order one off your own back though!
- May be used for retrobulbar haemorrhage (see p. 242).

CT and tumours

- Most imaging requests for tumour assessment come from registrar or consultant level, but there are some basics you should know.
- For tumour staging CT shows bony and cartilage invasion well, but MRI shows soft tissues better. MRI also shows marrow invasion (CT is poor).

- Tongue and floor-of-mouth cancers tend to be staged with MRI, although CT may be necessary to assess mandible invasion.
- Sino-nasal cancers need CT for the same reason.
- Laryngeal invasion is imaged best with CT.
- Many centres use CT to stage the neck (metastases), but MRI is usually better.
- Staging the chest and upper abdomen with CT is common with many head and neck cancers (up to 10% of head and neck cancers can have a synchronous primary tumour somewhere else in the aerodigestive system).

CT and infections

- You will need a contrast-enhanced CT which has a high sensitivity but low specificity.
- Imaging should be from skull base to carina because of the risk of mediastinitis.
- Usually looking for parapharyngeal, retropharyngeal, and submandibular spaces.
- The patient will have to lie flat which can make a bad airway worse, so make sure they are safe to go in the machine—airway loss in the scanner is a disaster. Don't be afraid to defer the decision up the chain of command. Patients are more easily seen in a CT than MRI (latter has a tunnel) and are more easily reached in an emergency situation.

Other uses of CT in OMFS

- CT angiograms for vascular malformations and assessment vessels in potential free flaps.
- Skull defect prior to reconstruction with cranioplasty. Can also assess skull vault thickness and presence of diploic space prior to calvarial bone graft harvesting.
- Assessment of complex craniofacial, developmental, or acquired deformity. 3D reconstruction is very helpful in these circumstances, and can be linked to a computer-assisted model, allowing the machine to visualize the problem even better.
- Large thyroid to assess retrosternal spread.
- For navigation-assisted surgery.
- For other surgery treatment planning such as stereolithographic models of the ilium for free-flap planning.
- For finding the source of a cerebrospinal fluid (CSF) leak.

Cone beam CT (CBCT)

General points

- Over the last decade CBCT has revolutionized imaging in OMFS.
- It is a relatively affordable technique which uses a single cone of radiation to give detailed image of small are such as the jaws.
- It uses less radiation than conventional CT.
- It is in danger of becoming over-used and exposing patients to excessive radiation to obtain an excellent image when actually a simple plain film would do, so beware—it's not a toy.

Uses of CBCT

- Better assessment of the relationship between the lower wisdom teeth and the inferior alveolar nerve (IAN) when plain film suggestive of intimate relationship *if* surgery is being considered. Another option is elective coronectomy, leaving the root behind.
- For planning implant placement, especially when close to the maxillary antrum or IAN. Assessment when alveolar ridge width is uncertain.
- TMJ pathology, fractures, or erosion.
- Intra-bony pathology, cysts/tumours/fibro-osseous lesions.
- To assess bony invasion of oral cancer.
- Facial deformity—often with a stereolithographic model.
- Assessment of unerupted teeth, probably only in complex cases.
- Assessment of airway space in obstructive sleep apnoea.
- Its role in trauma has yet to be fully established, but it is probably useful for zygomatic, complex, and orbital fractures as well as condylar neck fractures.
- It may also be useful for finding foreign bodies in the head and neck.

MRI and nuclear imaging

MRI and OMFS

- The most common use of MRI in OMFS is staging of malignancy.
- It is useful for parotid tumours where US cannot show the deep extent of a tumour because of the ramus of the mandible.
- MR sialograms are becoming a useful alternative to conventional sialography. They demonstrate more of the gland structure and do not use any radiation, but they have no therapeutic effect.
- For TMJ disc displacement MRI can be used to assess whether the disc is irreducibly displaced, and some experts believe that they can assess disc morphology.
- MR angiography can be used in the same way as CT angiography for vascular lesions and assessing blood flow for free-flap planning.
- In looking for causes of facial pain it may be used looking for SOL in brain, skull base or infratemporal fossa.
- MRI is very sensitive for diagnosis of osteomyelitis and also for assessing marrow involvement in tumour staging.

PET and OMFS

- Positron emission tomography (PET) of the head and neck region is usually used in combination with CT (PET-CT). This uses [^{18}F] deoxyglucose which is taken up by metabolically active cells. This unstable substance is made in a cyclotron, usually at the site of PET-CT or couriered in when needed. Therefore it is expensive!
- PET can show recurrent malignant disease in areas where it is difficult to examine such as the skull base, under flaps, or the tongue base.
- PET has a high false-positive rate but is very sensitive.
- After radiation you must wait about 3 months as the inflammation from the radiotherapy creates a false hot spot.
- Most PET-CTs are requested at senior level in special cases or for research. Few units use them routinely.

Sialography

General points

- Involves cannulation and subsequent injection of contrast medium into the gland ductal system and films taken at intervals thereafter.
- Three phases of sialography:
  - preoperative phase—scout film looking for radio-opaque stone.
  - filling phase—medium injected and films taken.
  - emptying phase: after ~5min a final film is taken of the gauge rate of emptying.
- Can be used with plain films or CT.
- Shows internal structure of the parotid or submandibular glandular systems.
- Can show strictures, stones (sialoliths), and dilatations (sialectasia).
- Some inference can be made about the dynamics of the system from rate of emptying.
- The 'pruned tree' appearance of the internal structure of the parotid gland as seen on the sialogram can point towards Sjögren's disease.
- Occasionally a salivary gland tumour may be apparent as rarely the first sign of the tumour is obstruction.
- The injection of a contrast agent may have a therapeutic effect, especially in patients with mucus plugging.
- MR sialography is an alternative.

In the emergency department

OMFS in the emergency department

A significant proportion of OMFS routine work is carried out in the ED under local anaesthesia. Therefore many patients can be seen, treated, and discharged home by the OMFS trainee.

Tips for success

- Be prepared. Bear in mind that some emergency units are woefully under-equipped for the full range of OMFS procedures, so take it upon yourself to organize an OMFS cupboard or trolley stocked with all the essentials: fine suture kits, absorbable/non-absorbable suture materials, local anaesthetic (dental syringes are finer and kinder to the patient if you can find them), dental splinting materials, bridle-wiring kits, gauze, Steri-Strips™, chloramphenicol ointment, microbiology swabs, and anything else you may need at arms' length.
- Escape the hubbub. Try to find a quiet room or area, with a good light source to perform examinations and minor procedures.
- Don't be afraid to ask for an assistant. There may be a willing nurse or trainee happy to put on some gloves to hand you equipment or cut sutures etc. An assistant can retract soft tissues, improve access, and cut sutures, as well as providing extra support if your patient is difficult to manage, particularly if they are under the influence of alcohol.
- Develop your skills. Many OMFS juniors resent being seen as a facial 'suture service' for A&E, but try to see it as an opportunity to enhance your surgical skills. Think about reconstruction, aesthetics, and healing, and take an interest in your work by following up the patients to see if a different approach may produce better results. This will benefit you further down the line if you choose to undertake higher surgical training.

Trauma patients and OMFS

Approach all patients referred to OMFS with an open mind. It may be a facial complaint that has prompted an OMFS referral, but there are often other injuries. Do not assume that these have already been dealt with by the A&E assessment. If you have any doubts, make it known to the referring emergency doctor. From an OMFS point of view, every trauma patient should be assessed using an advanced trauma life support (ATLS) approach. If a head injury is suspected, or there is a history of loss of consciousness, the patient must be examined and investigated by A&E before being deemed fit for discharge. If the patient requires admission for neurological observation, they should remain under the care of the emergency or trauma team until fit for discharge from a neurological point of view. For patients with polytrauma, early liaison with radiology is required to ensure that CT scans of the whole face, including mandible, are included, as if this is not requested at the time of admission or initial head CT, it can be difficult to organize later.

Admitting patients from A+E

Patients may be admitted if:
- they are systemically unwell
- they warrant observation overnight
- they require an operation under general anaesthesia (GA)
- there are concerns regarding their home support or social care

OMFS and alcohol consumption

- Alcohol and facial injuries go hand in hand.
- Be wary of patients who may have had a head injury If they are also drunk, signs of an intracranial injury may be disguised.
- Record carefully what the patient tells you regarding the history. If assault has been alleged, your notes will be used to produce a medical report for the police.

'Hospital dentist'

A significant proportion of A&E referrals will be for dental advice. Most OMFS departments do not want their juniors working as dentists in the ED and the ED will know the telephone numbers and hours of opening for local emergency dental services to discuss dental issues if required or advise patients accordingly, dental absesses are a different matter (📖 see p. 90).

The paediatric OMFS patient

- Facial and dental injuries are common in the paediatric patient. Always exclude more serious injury before dealing with the OMFS problem.
- Always examine in a paediatric department with a paediatric nurse.
- You may be lucky enough to have a paediatric dentist (📖 see p. 258) on site. If so, they will be an invaluable resource for dental injuries.

Deciduous dental injuries

- Re-implantation of avulsed teeth is NOT recommended in the primary dentition. All you need to do is account for the tooth.
- Subluxation (displaced) teeth can be left unless interfering with function (consider removal or manipulation (📖 see p. 199).
- Intruded teeth can often be left.
- Upper central incisors are the most commonly avulsed teeth. Adult central incisors appear at ~7 years of age.
- If a deciduous tooth has been injured, the patient should be warned that the permanent successor may be damaged and the general dental practitione (GDP) should be informed.
- 📖 See p. 88 for other tooth injuries.

Non-accidental injury and abuse

Unfortunately, a high index of suspicion is required. Facial injuries occur in many children suffering abuse, but will also occur in non-abused children.

- Injuries of different ages are suspicious.
- Cartilaginous structures may be deformed from repeated injury.
- Frenal tears in the very young and lacerations on the hard palate may indicate objects being forced into the mouth.
- Neglect may be heralded by multiple carious teeth.
- Pharyngeal gonorrhea is an indication of sexual abuse.

Lacerations

- Skin: both parent and child will be concerned about permanent scarring so be sensitive.
  - Tissue glues and Steri-Strips work well if the wound edges can be easily opposed.
  - If a couple of stitches are required GA may be avoided if both parent and child are cooperative. Use a topical anaesthetic before injecting the skin (📖 see p. 192).
- Oral mucosa:
  - Most intra-oral injuries will heal spontaneously.
  - Tongue lacerations do not generally require suture. Sucking an ice cube can help control bleeding. A forked tongue or tip injury may need repair.
  - Falling with an object in the mouth (e.g. a toothbrush or pen) can result in pharyngeal trauma. This may implant bacteria into the parapharyngeal spaces, causing local abscess or tracking media-stinitis, both of which can be life threatening. If there is no foreign body, this can often be managed conservatively (discuss with a senior). Prophylactic antibiotics may be required. Parents must be told to bring the child back IMMEDIATELY if there is any

temperature, drooling, or difficulty in swallowing or breathing. Injuries which breach muscle will normally require suture.

Fractures

- Facial fractures are rare in children, but if present often involve the mandibular condyle. This can have a serious impact on mandibular growth, with hypoplasia on the affected side resulting in possible facial asymmetry and occlusal abnormalities.
- Make sure that you have a high index of suspicion and adequate radiographs.

Dental pain and infections

- Dental infections can spread quickly in children.
- GA may be required to examine the mouth properly.
- Have a low threshold for admission; a couple of doses of IV antibiotics may help the situation.

Oral infections

There are many types (📖 see p. 216). The most common complaints are:
- ulceration—aphthous ulcers, trauma, primary herpetic gingivostomatitis, hand, foot, and mouth disease, herpangina, varicella zoster (chicken pox), and infectious mononucleosis (glandular fever).
- acute pseudo-membranous candidiasis (thrush).

Facial and oral swellings

- Parotitis (mumps) is much less common now but bacterial infection can also cause painful swelling of the parotid gland.
- Abscess: usually (but not always) painful. Look for a discharging sinus.
- Lymph nodes: cervical, auricular, and parotid lymph nodes are often enlarged in children. Check the scalp and inside the ears and mouth for possible causes.
- Un-erupted teeth: a displaced tooth may be palpable in the buccal sulcus or palate.
- Mucocele: damaged minor salivary gland usually presents as a bluish swelling inside the lower lip or floor of mouth (ranula).
- Eruption cyst: a cyst over an emerging tooth will usually pop spontaneously.

Epiglottitis

Traditionally the preserve of ENT surgeons, this frightening condition must be recognized quickly before the airway is threatened.

Signs

Fever, tachycardia, tachypnoea, inability to swallow, drooling, change in cry or speaking voice (hot potato voice)

▶▶ Management

Do not try to examine or lay the patient flat. Alert seniors and arrange immediate transfer to theatre for intubation or surgical airway.

Foreign bodies

Small objects frequently disappear up noses. If you can't see, it don't go hunting—you'll only make it more difficult to find. GA may be required.

Overview of maxillofacial trauma

Maxillofacial trauma is one of the most common presenting complaints at A&E. At least half a million facial injuries occur annually in the UK according to the results of the 1997 National Facial Injuries Survey[1]. Assessment can often be difficult because of the presence of a cervical collar, gross soft tissue swelling, and an un-cooperative patient. Therefore a methodical approach must be used.

All major trauma should be managed using ATLS principles. Technically, evaluation of maxillofacial injuries comes under the secondary survey. However, certain patterns of injury can lead to airway compromise and must be picked up early.

- Bilateral mandible fractures—the tongue loses its anterior muscular anchorage. The patient may refuse to lie flat to prevent airway occlusion.
- Inhaled teeth or dentures.
- Midface fractures—the entire palate can drop backwards to obstruct the oropharynx.
- Brisk bleeding in the mouth may necessitate log rolling to prevent inhalation (see p. 238).
- Laryngeal trauma—a surgical airway may be required (see p. 208).

Examination of the patient with major facial trauma

- Establish your own routine for examination.
- If the patient is wearing a collar, you will need someone to hold the head in in-line traction while you remove the collar to examine the mouth and neck.
- It is not uncommon for injuries to be missed, so ideally the examination should be performed again at a later date.
- Clear the head and face of blood.
- Examine the entire face and scalp for lacerations, abrasions, and foreign bodies (e.g. road grit). The patient may need to be turned to examine the back of the head.
- Methodically palpate the cranium, not forgetting the mastoid processes, and bony ridges of the facial skeleton looking for boggy swellings, step deformities, and depressions.
- Assess for exo- or enophthalmus. This can be very difficult if there is a lot of swelling, but a tense bulging eye indicates a retrobulbar haemorrhage requiring immediate decompression (see p. 242). Check pupillary reflexes, eye movements, and visual acuity. Note any subconjunctival haemorrhage or trauma to the globe and eyelids.
- Feel the bridge of the nose. Is it widened, flattened, or deviated? Look up the nose (use a nasal speculum and suction) for septal haematoma, septal deviation, bleeding points, and CSF leak.
- Examine the pinna for lacerations. Clean the ear canal and perform otoscopy. Is there bleeding from behind the drum (a bulging purplish appearance)? Is it perforated? You must distinguish blood from the

1 Hutchison IL, Magennis P, Shepherd JP, Brown AE (1998). The BAOMS United Kingdom survey of facial injuries part 1: aetiology and the association with alcohol consumption. *British Journal of Oral and Maxillofacial Surgery* **36**: 3–13.

face pooling in the ear to blood coming from inside the ear, which is an important clinical sign, indicating base of skull fracture (ditto with CSF from the ear).

- Grasp the upper incisors and alveolus between finger and thumb and gently rock backwards and forwards to detect any movement (movement means fracture). Press on the face with your other hand whilst rocking the palate to assess the level of fracture (📖 see p. 75). Slide a finger up into each buccal sulcus feeling for bulges from zygomatic complex fractures.
- Look inside the mouth, noting lacerations, missing or damaged teeth, alveolar fractures, dentures (remove to prevent aspiration).
- Feel along the lower border of the mandible, assess mouth opening, and check for mobile segments and lacerations on the gingiva (📖 see p. 67).
- Look at the neck for swelling, bruising, and puncture wounds. Feel for airway deviation and surgical emphysema.
- Examine the cranial nerves.

Record your findings carefully. Not only will it help you to organize your investigations and treatment of complex injuries, but sometimes criminal proceedings follow an injury and you may be required to testify in court.

Investigations
- If the patient is having a CT head to exclude intracranial injury, discuss with the radiologist to ensure that the facial skeleton is included and that it is reformatted in the coronal plane.
- Remember that the patient will not be able to have facial X-rays until the c-spine is cleared, and a DPT will have to wait until the patient can stand up.

Thinking beyond the face
- Serious intracranial injury, cervical injury, pulmonary injury, and sight-threatening ocular injuries are not uncommon in severe maxillofacial trauma.[2] Early recognition of these injuries is key to improving outcome.
- Alcohol is often implicated in the aetiology of facial injuries[1]. Always ask for an alcohol history and prescribe appropriate medication if withdrawal is likely.
- Large numbers of women suffering domestic abuse will attend A&E with facial injuries. Sensitively ask about home life—an admission for social reasons may be necessary.

2 Alvi A, Doherty T, Lewen G (2003). Facial fractures and concomitant injuries in trauma patients. *Laryngoscope* **113**: 102–6.

Mandibular fractures

- Mandibular fractures are common, but do not underestimate the force taken to break a jaw. The mandible is the densest bone in the body so the cranium will have absorbed a considerable impact—always rule out significant head injury.
- As always, be mindful that swelling can develop, especially in the floor of mouth, and threaten the airway.
- Occasionally it can be difficult to detect a fracture. A good knowledge of the patterns of fractures will help direct you in examining the radiographs (see p. 69).
- Some isolated uncomplicated non-displaced fractures can be managed conservatively. Advise a soft diet and review in the clinic.
- Because of its shape the mandible often fractures in more than one place (most commonly parasymphysis and angle/condyle), so if you diagnose one fracture look for more.
- Anterior mandible fractures are commonly missed on radiographs because of the angle of the beam so make the diagnosis clinically.

History

The most common mechanism of injury is assault or road traffic accidents, although sports-related fractures are increasing. ♂ > ♀ and alcohol is implicated in up to 40%. Patients may describe hearing a crack on impact. Some ignore the injury until they wake up in the morning with a sore swollen face.

Symptoms

Difficulty in swallowing or breathing should ring alarm bells. Pain is variable and worsened by eating and talking. Swelling is also variable and can hinder examination. Patients describe their teeth not meeting together; this is not a reliable indicator of fracture as it can occur with bruising or joint effusion. However, paraesthesia of the lower teeth and lip is a good indicator of fracture and **must** be carefully documented to exclude later iatrogenic damage.

Signs

- **Posture**—patients often use their hands to support the fractured segment and may be unable to close fully, resulting in drooling.
- **Swelling** can be diffuse and extend into the submandibular space and down the neck.
- **Step deformity** on lower border of the mandible (may be difficult to assess).
- **Trismus** from swelling or condylar fracture.
- **Step in occlusion** or anterior/posterior open bites.
- **Mobile teeth**.
- **Gingival laceration/bruising** at the site of the stepped occlusion.
- **Sublingual haematoma**.
- **Paraesthesia** in distribution of the inferior dental nerve (IDN).
- **Compression test**—if the fracture is obvious there is no need to test for mobility. Gentle backward pressure on the point of the chin can provoke pain in angle of condylar fracture; likewise simultaneous medial pressure on the angles can reveal fractures of the symphyseal region.
- **Bite strength**—ask the patient to bite firmly on a cotton roll or tongue depressor. If you can't withdraw it from their teeth, chance of fractire is small.

NB: Bilateral symphyseal fractures mean that forward attachment of the tongue is lost and there is a danger of loss of airway from its backward displacement.

Radiographs (Fig. 4.1)

- Most commonly DPT plus PA mandible but lower occlusal views are also acceptable and give a good view of the anterior region (📖 see p. 42).
- Ensure that the entire condyles are both visible.
- Systematically trace the outline of the mandible, noting any discontinuity. Fractures often extend through the roots of teeth (i.e. where the bone is thinnest). Canines have the longest roots, so parasymphyseal fractures here are common.
- Angle fractures commonly involve 8s if present.
- Note the degree of displacement and comminution, and the prognosis of the teeth (i.e. are the teeth grossly carious?)
- CT is helpful for condylar fractures and complicated fractures.

Management

- Most fractures will need open reduction and internal fixation (ORIF) (📖 see p. 150). Some undisplaced fractures can be managed conservatively—discuss with your senior.

- Mandible fractures are usually open fractures, communicating with either the tooth socket or directly into the oral cavity. IV antibiotics (e.g. benzylpenicillin and metronidazole) are indicated.
- Admit the patient, place on the emergency list, and work up for theatre (preoperative bloods etc.), analgesia, IV fluids, and nil by mouth (NBM).
- Simple bridle wiring of mobile segments can relieve pain (◫ see p. 201). Take impressions if custom-made arch bars will be needed (e.g condylar fractures, multiple fractures).
- You must be adequately trained to take consent. The important points are listed in Box 4.1.

Special circumstances

- Children often fall onto chin and will not open mouth. Condylar intracapsular fractures are common, result in intense pain, and are un-detectable on plain X-ray. Review in clinic and request CBCT
- Guardsman fracture—fall onto chin in adult resulting in bilateral condylar head fracture and midline symphysis fracture. So called because the injury is found in soldiers who faint while on guard duty.

Box 4.1 Points to note when obtaining consent

- Fractures are fixed with plates and screws; occasionally inter-maxillary fixation (IMF; jaw wiring) is required. They may need elastics (small rubber bands) postoperatively.
- The approach is usually intra-oral, but sometimes very small incisions need to be made on the face to gain access.
- Teeth with a poor prognosis may have to be extracted.
- There will be postoperative swelling and trismus,
- Numb lip ± tongue is common postoperatively. There is a small chance of lasting paraesthesia, usually when the nerve has been severely damaged by the trauma.

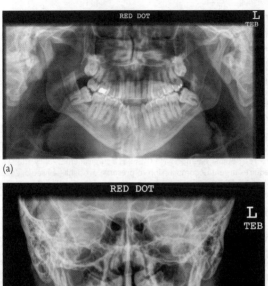

(a)

(b)

Fig. 4.1 (a) OPG showing displaced right parasymphyseal fracture and non-displaced left low condyle fracture. (b) PA mandible showing the same patient, note how the left condylar fracture is almost invisible on the PA view.

Zygomatic fractures

- Most fractures occur at the junction of the zygoma with other bones (i.e. orbit and maxilla) and so are probably best termed 'zygomatic complex fractures'.
- The classic fracture pattern cause by a direct blow to the prominence of the check is the **tripod fracture** with disruption of the zygomatico-frontal suture, depression of the zygomatic arch, and fracture of the infraorbital rim. Some argue that there is a fourth fracture of the zygomatic buttress, which is commonly buckled.
- It can be a challenge to assess these fractures because of the marked periorbital swelling.
- Very rarely there is an indication for immediate action, but ▶▶retrobulbar haemorrhage (RBH) is a surgical emergency and requires urgent decompression to preserve eyesight (📖 see p. 242).
- Always fully assess eyes and record results of the Snellen chart in the notes (a handy copy is on the inside back cover of this book).

Signs

There is usually a cosmetic ± functional problem
- **Loss of prominence of the cheek**—best examined from behind the patient looking down onto the face.
- **Zygomatico-frontal (ZF) tenderness**—palpation over the ZF suture (upper outer corner of the orbit) can reveal a step deformity.
- **Step in the infraorbital rim or zygomatic arch**.
- **Subconjunctival haemorrhage**—if the posterior limit cannot be identified, this suggests orbital wall fracture.
- **Buttress fracture**—this is examined intraorally by sliding a finger along the buccal sulcus above the upper molars. Bruising may be visible in the mucosa.
- **Trismus**—the depressed arch impinges the mandibular condyle (can be confused with mandible fracture).
- **Infraorbital nerve paraesthesia**—usually a neuropraxia injury as it exits the infraorbital foramen, resulting in variable altered sensation to the cheek, side of nose and upper lip. This can also occur in the absence of fracture.
- **Unilateral epistaxis**—overflow from the maxillary sinus as it fills up with blood.
- **Eye injuries**—the globe is relatively protected by the orbit, but depending on the mechanism of injury a range of injuries are possible. You must fully examine the eye and refer to Ophthalmology if there are any concerns.

❶ Always remember to check that the maxilla is stable to avoid missing a Le Fort fracture.

Investigations

Radiographs

Two OM views (📖 see p. 48). Complex fractures require CT with 3D reformatting. Assess the films systematically.

- Campbell's lines—follow a line across both zygomatic arches and another line through both coronoid processes across the maxillary antrum and base of nose.
- Look at the ZF suture and compare with the other side to detect widening.
- Check the distance between the coronoid process and the lower border of the arch on each side. It will be reduced in a fracture.
- Fluid levels can sometimes be seen in the maxillary antrum, but this can also occur in the absence of a fracture (e.g from a nosebleed or even a cold).

Management

- Any eye problems should be referred to Ophthalmology (except RBH which you should manage expectantly and then refer).
- Some surgeons advocate immediate surgical reduction of displaced zygoma fractures. However, most units review a fracture in clinic in 5–7 days and if surgery is indicated plan this for about 2 weeks post injury when swelling has lessened and therefore adequate reduction can be assessed on the operating table (📖 see p. 154).
- ❶ Always inform the patient **not** to blow their nose—this can result in surgical emphysema from the maxillary sinus and upper respiratory tract bacteria are implanted directly into the tissues. Tell them they may well get some blood from the nose, but that they should only wipe.
- For the same reason antibiotics should be considered. Some consultants routinely like their zygoma fracture patients to have antibiotics, while others do not. Make sure that you know your local protocol.
- Warn them that diplopia may improve *or* get worse as the swelling resolves (📖 see p. 113).

How to assess the eye

- Ask about diplopia, painful eye, nose bleeds.
- **Look** for swelling, exo/enophthalmus (posterior displacement of globe), hypoglobus (downward displacement), subconjunctival haemorrhage.
- **Feel**—assess how tense the globe is. There should be some give—feel your own.
- **Visual acuity**—ideally a full sized Snellen chart at 3m. Often a mirror is used to double the distance (i.e. at 1.5m). You must record an objective figure (e.g. 3/3).
- **Reflexes**—red, direct, and consensual (in RBH direct is lost but consensual remains).
- **Fields**—check all movements and record any subjective diplopia and objective restriction in movement.
- **Fundoscopy and slit lamp examination**—this may not be needed if the patient is to be reviewed by Ophthalmology, but it is good practice to check inside the eye. Cells within the anterior chamber can be identified fairly easily.

Eye examination is often complicated by the patient's inability to open the eyelid because of swelling. Check that they can perceive light through the lid and look for a consensual reflex in the unaffected eye.

Orbital floor fractures

- Orbital fractures occur as part of zygomatic complex fractures or as isolated orbital floor fractures—**blow-out fracture**.
- Seven bones join to form the orbit, five of which make up the orbital floor—zygoma, maxilla, palatine, ethmoidal, and lacrimal (the other two are greater wing of sphenoid and frontal).
- The outer rim of the orbit is thick, but the orbital floor becomes very thin particularly posteriomedially, and hence this is where fractures are most likely to be found. The teleological argument for this 'design' is that fractures occur to prevent damage to structures of the globe when orbital volume is suddenly increased (e.g by a blow to the eye).
- The following structures can be involved in floor fractures.
  - *Inferior orbital fissure*—contains the maxillary nerve and its zygomatic branch and branches of the pterygopalantine ganglion (parasympathetic to lacrimal gland).
  - *Infraorbital canal*—contains the infraorbital nerve and vessels and runs under the middle of the orbital floor.
- Most fractures are medial to the infraorbital canal (the optic canal is superior and relatively protected).

Orbital floor fractures are usually a result of a direct blow to the eye. Often there is gross swelling and bruising, although sometimes a fracture may be associated with a complete absence of signs.

RBH, although rare (0.3%), usually occurs with a zygomatic fracture. However, always think of it as a possibility with any circumorbital trauma.

Signs

- **Diplopia**—it is important to distinguish whether this is due to entrapment of the tissues in the fracture (which can be improved by surgery) or nerve injury causing muscle dysfunction (managed conservatively). Diagnosis is by orthoptic assessment.
- **Enophthalmos** is due to an increase in the volume of the orbit, most noticeable with fractures behind the globe.
- **Hypoglobus**—check the interpupillary line.
- **Subconjunctival haemorrhage**—when extending distally, this suggests orbital wall fracture.
- **Tenderness/step of infraorbital rim**.
- **Infraorbital nerve parasthesia**.

▶▶ Orbital injuries in children

The springy orbital floor entraps periorbital tissues like a trap door. There is no subconjunctival haemorrhage, so this is called the **white eye blow-out**. The trapped tissue causes acute pain and restriction in upward gaze, and can be seen as a shadow hanging down into the maxillary sinus radiographically—'teardrop sign'. The oculo-cardiac reflex can be pronounced in children, with afferent vagal stimulation resulting in brady-cardia, hypotension, and vomiting.

❶ Urgent surgical intervention is required to prevent muscle necrosis. All children should be followed up long-term by ophthalmic surgeons after release of the trap.

Radiology (Fig. 4.2)

OM views can show a fluid level in the sinus and herniation of tissue but visualization of the fracture site (i.e. if for surgical repair) will require CT with coronal reformatting

Management

- Always admit any child.
- All orbital floor fractures should have ophthalmic surgery review—you should discuss with the on-call doctor. They may elect to see in clinic if visual acuity is not affected (see p. 113).
- Arrange for a Hess chart and binocular visual orthoptic assessment if there is any diplopia or restricted movement (as an outpatient for adults)
- Review in clinic in 3–5 days to assess whether surgery is indicated (obtain CT orbits if you think this is likely).
- Instruct patients not to blow their nose, as with zygoma fractures, and to return to A&E if they experience further eye pain. Consider antibiotics.
- Swollen eyes can be kept clean with sterile water and cotton wool plus chloramphenicol ointment (1%).

Indications for surgical repair

- **Absolute**—muscle entrapment, especially in young patients.
- **Relative**—significant increase in orbital volume likely to result in hypoglobus, enophthalmus, and diplopia. The surgical dilemma is that diplopia can occur several months later when repair of fracture is difficult. Hence pre-emptive treatment might be required.

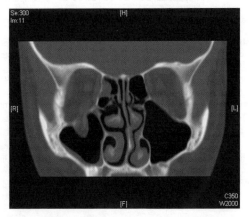

Fig 4.2 Coronal reformatted CT scan of the orbits showing a right orbital floor fracture with herniation of the periorbital fat and inferior rectus muscle.

Maxillary fractures

- Midface fractures occur along lines of weakness, resulting in the patterns described by Rene Le Fort in 1901 (Fig. 4.3).
- These are less common than mandibular and zygomatic fractures but can involve both in pan-facial injuries.
- The level of fracture might not be the same on both sides and sometimes is incomplete.
- Frequently these fractures are associated with major trauma, so check for c-spine and head injury.
- When craniomaxillary dysjunction occurs (the bones of the face literally come off the skull), the mobile segment can displace posteriorly and obstruct the airway. It needs to be disimpacted immediately.
- Associated laceration of the maxillary artery can result in brisk bleeding, compounding difficulty in securing the airway (📖 see p. 238).

History

Typically there is a history of major trauma e.g RTA but occasionally a Le Fort 1 fracture can be induced from a minor fall in an elderly edentulous patient wearing an upper denture.

Signs

- **Horse face/dish face**—the facial skeleton slides backwards and downwards on the skull base, retruding and lengthening it.
- **Posterior gagging**—back teeth meet prematurely due to posterior displacement of maxilla with resultant **anterior open bite**.
- **Bilateral black eyes** (NB: must exclude base skull fracture) and subconjunctival haemorrhage.
- **Palatal haematoma** (can signify midline palatal fracture) and bruising in the buccal sulcus and soft palate
- **Mobility of palatal segment** and cracked cup resonance on tapping upper teeth. In midline palatal fractures the upper teeth show mobility on compression across the arch.

Always look for CSF leak indicating associated cribiform plate fracture (signs of this are 'tram-lining' of blood in fluid from the nose or a 'target' spot of blood on the pillow, and can be checked by sending a sample for β-transferrin measurement).

Radiology

- Plain films used for diagnosis are the OM views and lateral cephalogram. The X-rays are systematically examined using the lines described by Campbell and McGregor.
- Complex fractures will require CT with coronal/3D reformatting.

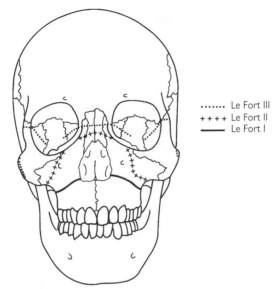

······ Le Fort III
+ + + + Le Fort II
——— Le Fort I

Fig. 4.3 Le Fort diagram. Reproduced from Mitchell L, Mitchell D, *Oxford Handbook of Clinical Dentistry* (5th edn), p.461 (Oxford: 2009). With permission from Oxford University Press.

Management

- Usually these patients will require admission because of associated injuries. Repair can be complex when there are many comminuted segments and is probably best left until the swelling is resolved. Custom-made arch bars can be used, so take some impressions. (This might be a bit tricky when the maxilla is very mobile!)

Occasionally isolated maxillary fractures can be managed conservatively with a Gunning splint (a type of modified denture).

Nose, naso-ethmoidal, and frontal bone fractures

Fractured nose

- Nasal fractures are exceedingly common. They often do not need treatment unless the patient complains of a functional or cosmetic problem.
- Examine the nose from above and behind, although deviation may be difficult to detect because of swelling. In severe fractures try to use some local anaesthetic spray before examining inside the nose. Plain films are not needed to diagnose nasal fracture, although OM views may be used to rule out associated facial injury.
- Epistaxis can be impressive and may require packing (📖 see p. 238). Do not let it divert your attention from ruling out two important negatives.
  - Head injury—bilateral black eyes are associated with nasal fracture but can also be a sign of skull base fracture.
  - Septal haematoma—use a good light and nasal speculum to examine the septum. If it is purple, shiny and bulging you need to evacuate using a scalpel to prevent cartilage necrosis. You must document that you have checked for this.
- Some advocate manipulating and realigning the nasal bones immediately using the lateral surfaces of both your thumbs to provide traction, or forceps if you happen to have some to hand. This will be eye-wateringly painful for your patient, but may save them a GA. Do not attempt it if you have not been shown how!
- Any patients requiring treatment should be reviewed in clinic in 5–7 days where decision to perform manipulation under anaesthesia (MUA) can be made (📖 see p. 116).

Naso-ethmoidal fracture

- This rare injury is caused by significant blunt trauma across the bridge of the nose and is often associated with a contusion or laceration in this region.
- There is a characteristic appearance in profile with flattening of the bridge of the nose, which has an upturned tip (think Peter Pan).
- Traumatic telecanthus increase in distance between the medial canthi is caused by loss of medial attachment of the canthi to the nasal bones and can be difficult to correct. Measure the intercanthal distance, which would normally be half the interpupillary distance, and record both these figures in the notes.
- Other signs include periorbital ecchymosis and telescoping of the nasal bones.
- Clean and suture any associated lacerations and obtain detailed 3D CT scans. Surgical treatment can be performed on a semi-elective basis.

Frontal bone fracture

- Essentially this is caused by the same mechanism as for naso-ethmoidal fractures but just a few centimetres higher, often with an overlying laceration.
- The underlying frontal sinus is highly variable in size and morphology, which can complicate diagnosis of fracture from plain films. A history of significant injury in this region requires a CT scan.
- Frontal sinus fractures can be either:
  - Anterior wall—depressed fracture will result in poor cosmesis. You may be able to feel a bony step through the forehead wound.
  - Posterior wall—when displaced by more than its thickness there is likely to be an associated dural tear. These are treated surgically (by cranialization of the sinus and obliteration of the fronto-nasal duct) to prevent later complications such as meningitis, brain abscess, and mucopyocele.
- Clean and suture any lacerations and prescribe antibiotics.[1]

1 Yavuzer R et al. (2005) Management of frontal sinus fractures, *Plastic and Reconstructive Surgery* **115**: 79e–93e.

Face and scalp soft tissue injuries

Tips for success

- Mechanism of injury is important to consider.
- Wounds should generally be closed within 24 hours.
- Good light for examination and treatment.
- Always look for an underlying bony injury.
- Don't forget associated structures that could be involved, including blood vessels, nerves, ducts or glands (📖 see p. 26).
- Achieve haemostasis with local pressure or bipolar diathermy if required.
- Functional outcome and aesthetics are of utmost importance when planning and performing treatment—try to minimize scarring.
- A compliant patient is mandatory. If the patient is too drunk to deal with, wash the wound, dress it, and arrange to suture when the patient has sobered up.
- Stick within your means—if complex reconstruction is required, discuss with senior.

History and assessment

History

Take a thorough history including the time and mechanism of injury. Blunt or penetrating trauma? Has a weapon been used? Was broken glass involved? Is there likely to be head injury, c-spine injury, or fractures to the facial skeleton? Medical history, social history, and tetanus status.

Examination

Carefully inspect the face and scalp. Record all soft tissue injuries on a diagram, including location, size, and nature of all wounds. Diagrams are good.

Investigations

If there is any chance of broken glass in the wound, take a soft tissue radiograph (discuss with radiographers)—most glass and inorganic material is radio-opaque (📖 see p. 49).

Types of wound

Laceration

- **Straight**—close in layers. Try to evert the edges with skin sutures to aid healing and use minimum sutures to re-appose the edges nicely.
- **Shelved**—consider excising the shelved area to make the wound edges appose at right angles. Thin sections of skin can often 'retract', giving the appearance of a worse injury. Ensure that the retracted skin is replaced in its original position.
- **Crush**—gently squeeze out haematoma or congealed blood. Minimally excise any contused or ragged wound edges. Light skin apposition. Can often be swollen.

Abrasion

The epidermis is removed by friction and the dermis is left exposed. This will granulate and heal nicely if thoroughly cleaned, debrided, and dressed with chloramphenicol or white soft paraffin to keep clean.

Beware of 'tattooing'—grit or dirt literally forced into the tissues by high frictional forces. These wounds must be scrubbed vigorously to lift the grit and prevent permanent marks on the skin/underlying tissues. Perform under GA if a large surface area is affected.

Bite injuries

These are commonly dog bites, but cat bites and human bites are also seen. Cat and human bites are particularly prone to developing infection. Animal bites to the face are more common in children.[1] Thorough, early washout of these wounds is required. Bite wounds are usually polymicrobially contaminated, so give co-amoxiclav prophylaxis for 5–7 days. Give a tetanus booster and consider human tetanus immunoglobulin (if the wound is highly contaminated or the patient is immunosuppressed). It is possible that viruses can be transmitted via human bites, although the risk is likely to be very small. A risk assessment of the biter should be made and, if appropriate, hepatitis B vaccine/immunoglobulin and/or HIV post-exposure prophylaxis should be offered. Bite wounds can be closed primarily if thoroughly cleaned, but if in doubt consider delayed closure.[2]

Anatomical areas—specific tips

Eyebrow/forehead

Preserve the eyebrow's shape and form. Repair underlying frontalis muscle to prevent spreading and further depression of scar. Only minimum debridement of ragged wound edges should be performed—conservation of skin on the forehead is a priority to minimize contracture. Scar revision can be performed at a later date if necessary.

Eyelid

Unless the injuries are superficial, get help—margin involvement or muscle injury needs expert repair. Rule out penetrating injury to the globe. Use fine sutures left long and Steri-Stripped to the side to prevent sharp suture ends from catching the eye. If the patient is unable to elevate the eyelid, there could be an injury to levator palpebrae superioris. This needs early repair—refer to senior.

Lacrimal

The lacrimal gland and ducts are located superior and lateral to the upper lid margin, The draining superior and inferior canaliculi leading to the lacrimal duct are located in the medial corner of the eye, above and below the medial canthus. If you suspect injury, DO NOT attempt to close, as careful repair under a microscope is needed.

1 Weiss HB, Friedman DI, Coben JH (1998). Incidence of dog bite injuries treated in emergency departments. Journal of the *American Mdical Association*, **279**: 51–3.
2 Stefanopoulos PK, Tarantzopoulou AD. Facial bite wounds: management update. *International Journal of Oral and Maxillofacial Surgery* **34**: 464–72.

Ears

Exclude and/or drain any perichondral haematoma to prevent a cauliflower ear from developing—repair in layers, use pressure dressing, and review. Debride ear wounds conservatively. If cartilage sutures are required, use prolene 5'0. Never leave exposed cartilage. Prescribe post-operative co-amoxiclav. For complicated lacerations or ear avulsion injuries, call a senior.

Nose

Ensure that the nostril borders are re-aligned. If the wound is deep through the nasal mucosa, close the mucosa first with absorbable 4'0 sutures and then the skin with 5'0 sutures. Nasal cartilage should be repositioned by closing the mucosa and skin over it. A nostril splint can be used.

Cheeks

Rule out injury to the parotid duct/gland and facial nerve. Ensure that thorough testing of facial nerve is completed before infiltrating with local anaesthesia (LA). If the nerve damage is medial to the lateral canthal line, the facial nerve is probably unrepairable.

If the wound involves the gland but not the duct, you can repair the gland in A&E, taking care to re-suture the parotid fascia to avoid development of a sialocoele. If a ductal or facial nerve injury is suspected, the patient must be taken to theatre for a formal exploration and repair within 72 hours.

Mouth/lips

The priority is to re-approximate the vermillion border to avoid a 'step' upon healing. Labial mucosa and orbicularis oris should also be precisely apposed and closed with a resorbable suture. Through-and-through lacerations should be closed in layers. Good OH and salt rinses post-operatively aid healing (📖 see p. 177).

Penetrating injuries to the neck

- Penetrating neck trauma may involve a sharp object or missile that has penetrated the skin and underlying platysma. This may include puncture wounds, stabbing injuries, gunshot wounds, or impalement.
- A penetrating injury to the neck can potentially inflict massive damage to the internal structures that run through the neck and result in catastrophic airway, vascular, or neurological injuries.
- Therefore a seemingly small innocuous wound to the skin of the neck can present a threat to the patient's life.
- The neck can be thought of in zones of potential damage (Fig. 4.4).[1]
  - **Zone I**—inferior aspect of cricoid cartilage to the thoracic outlet. Contains proximal common carotid artery, vertebral artery, subclavian artery, internal jugular vein (and subclavian vein which sometimes comes above the clavicle), trachea, oesophagus, thoracic duct (left side) and thymus.
  - **Zone II**—cricoid to angle of mandible. Contains internal/external carotid arteries, jugular veins, pharynx, larynx, oesophagus, recurrent laryngeal nerve, spinal cord, trachea, thyroid and parathyroid glands.
  - **Zone III**—angle of mandible to the base of skull. Contains distal extra-cranial carotid and vertebral arteries, internal carotid, and jugular vein and its tributaries.
- Management may be observational (if patient is stable), surgical exploration ± adjunctive invasive or non-invasive management.

Clinical features

- Dysphagia
- Hoarseness
- Oro/nasopharyngeal bleeding
- Neurological defect
- Hypotension
- Subcutaneous emphysema
- Stridor
- Haematoma with neck swelling
- Bruit/thrill
- Pulselessness

Initial management

ATLS approach—primary and secondary survey.

- **A** To secure a definitive airway, endotracheal intubation may be required. Get senior anaesthetic help. An emergency cricothyroidotomy may be indicated if unable to intubate through the vocal cords. If the trachea has been lacerated, intubation through the wound may be a lifesaving action, although this would probably be necessary long before the patient gets to hospital.
- **B** Ensure adequate oxygenation and that both lungs have normal air entry.

The zones of the neck

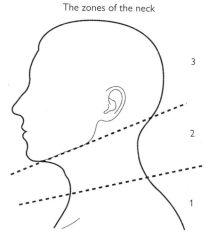

Fig. 4.4 Zones of the neck in relation to penetrating injuries. Reproduced from Banghu A, Lee C, and Porter K, *Emergencies in Trauma*, p.30 (Oxford: 2010). With permission from Oxford University Press.

- **C** The priority is to get local control of bleeding. Replacing dressings won't work. A finger stuck into the neck wound may be the only way to control arterial bleeding. Haemostats or artery clips can be used for visible bleeding vessels. Bilateral wide-bore IV access. Fluid resuscitate, although not too aggressively, as the increase in blood pressure may make matters worse in severe bleeding effort is made to do C at the same time as A, and the BATLS before.

Possible investigations (discuss with senior)
- Full blood count (FBC), group and save (G&S), cross-match.
- Cervical AP and lateral radiograph.
- Chest X-ray (CXR)—pneumothorax.
- Conventional angiography—for external carotid bleeding. It may even be possible to embolize the vessel at this time.
- Doppler duplex ultrasonography.
- Barium swallow.
- CT—helical or spiral CT permits multiplanar views and 3D reconstructions. Good for laryngeal injuries.
- CT angiography (CTA)—replacing angiography as initial study of choice for suspected vascular injury.
- MRI—not routinely used as it takes too long.
- MR angiography (MRA)—time constraints limit use.
- Direct laryngoscopy.
- Flexible bronchoscopy.

- Oesophagoscopy—risk of perforation into neck and introduction of bacteria into neck spaces because of gas insufflation used at the time of procedure.

Definitive management

After primary survey and resuscitation:
- observation or expectant management for those who are stable;
- consider further investigations (only if stable);
- immediate exploration for patients with ongoing signs and symptoms of shock or continued haemorrhage.

Reference

1 Biffl WL *et al.* (1997). Selective management of penetrating neck trauma based on cervical level of injury. *American Journal of Surgery* **174**: 678–82.

Intra-oral injuries

Overview

- Intra-oral trauma is common in children, particularly toddlers who have a tendency to run and play with objects in the mouth.
- Good blood supply and the properties of saliva means that both injuries and incisions in the mouth generally heal quickly.
- Intra-oral changes may manifest secondary to bony fractures of the mandible or maxilla.
- Anatomy. (📖 see p. 12)

Anatomical areas

Soft palate, tonsil and posterior pharynx.

- Injuries to these areas are relatively common as they are directly posterior to the opening of the mouth.
- Penetrating injures can be caused by falling onto a sharp object (particularly toddlers) or stabbing injuries—accidental or otherwise.
- Wounds can look innocuous on examination (small puncture wound), but neurological or vascular injury could occur if the object has penetrated deep enough.
- Potentially close to internal carotid, cranial nerves IX, X, and XII, sympathetic plexus, and internal jugular vein.
- Consider liaising with ENT. May require GA and exploration.
- Often managed conservatively.

Tongue

- Lacerations—if located on the dorsum of the tongue, can normally be managed conservatively. If on lateral border or tip, should be sutured to prevent fissured healing.
- Tongue studs can become infected and swell to a phenomenal size. May be risk to airway. Management is to remove the stud and prescribe antibiotics. Studs placed laterally can damage the lingual artery!

Lips

- Careful approximation of the vermilion border is required (make this the first 'marking' stitch to avoid an uneven pull from stitches on either side)
- Full-thickness lip lacerations should have layered closure after washout and debridement
- Beware of the labial arteries—if cut and not tied off or coagulated with diathermy can produce significant labial haematoma or bleeding. They also bleed from both ends!

Gingivae

- Torn gingivae may mean that there is a fracture of the maxilla/mandible or alveolar bone

De-gloving injuries of lower jaw

- Essentially this occurs when the soft tissues have been ripped off the mandible by blunt trauma.
- These are dirty wounds and require copious irrigation and closure under GA.
- They can often be missed at examination if the tissues are stuck down.

Teeth

📖 See p. 10.

General intra-oral injury management

- Small wounds do not usually require surgical intervention and will heal quickly.
- Salt mouth rinses aid healing and reduce infection risk. Make sure you tell the patient they must clean their teeth as normal with a brush and paste.
- If the wound is dirty and contaminated, antibiotic prophylaxis can be considered.
- Intra-oral wounds will initially look yellow and sloughy when healing—this does not mean that they are infected.
- Patients with deeper penetrating injuries should be monitored for neurological or vascular signs.
- Foreign bodies—identify with radiographs if possible. Ultrasound (US) may also be useful here, particularly for radiolucent objects (such as wood).
- Stitching in the mouth—use absorbable sutures and think about knot placement to increase comfort for patient.
- Through-and-through wounds need careful closure in layers to prevent oro-cutaneous/salivary fistula.

Non-accidental injury (NAI)

Perioral injuries are very common in children when they fall or bump into things at face height. Intra-oral injuries are less common, but do occur accidentally. Look out for fraenal tears and palatal injuries, which can occur secondary to objects being forced into mouths. Always take a detailed history of what happened and examine the area in question as well as the rest of the body. If in any doubt about the cause of the injury, discuss with a senior (and involve the paediatric team who are trained in recognition and management of NAI).

Dento-alveolar trauma

It can be difficult to manage trauma to teeth in A&E because of the lack of equipment and dental radiographs. Do the best you can to stabilize the injuries until the patient can be assessed and treated by their dentist or in the dental hospital.

Check that fragments have not been inhaled (may need CXR) or lost into the soft tissues.

Replace avulsed teeth as soon as you can. This is a dental emergency as the chances of saving the tooth rapidly decrease with the amount of time that it has spent out of the mouth (see p. 199).

Severely intruded or displaced teeth and fractures of the alveolar bone necessitate follow-up by OMFS. The rest can be managed by the dentist (many patients are not registered with a GDP which can complicate matters).

Make sure that you achieve good anaesthesia before examining the mouth. Most injuries will be 'luxation injuries' (loosening). The tooth may not be wobbly *per se*, but there will have been some damage to the periodontal ligament holding the tooth in its socket.

Tooth fracture

Crown fracture

Simple fracture of enamel ± dentine. It has a good prognosis and is best managed by the GDP. Sensitivity can be avoided by sealing any exposed dentine with bonding agent. Check the lip for intruded fragments (soft tissue X-ray helps).

Complicated fracture

Fractures which expose the pulp will usually require root canal treatment (RCT). The situation is complicated in children where the root apex is incompletely formed. The exposed nerve will be acutely painful, so dress it (you may need to inject LA into the pulp). CaOH or ledermix can be directly applied and a temporary filling material added on top.

Root fracture

Splinting + RCT is the mainstay of treatment. Fractures of the coronal 3rd have the worst prognosis and may best be treated by decoronation and crowning (see p. 258).

Luxation injuries

Concussion/subluxation

A certain amount of force can be absorbed by the periodontal ligament, meaning that the tooth is not grossly displaced. Essentially these two injuries are the same, but are clinically differentiated as a subluxed tooth has blood around the gingival margin. The tooth can be very tender so a soft diet is recommended. The tooth should be monitored by the GDP as pulpal necrosis can occur and result in a discoloration of the tooth.

Lateral luxation/intrusion/extrusion

In these injuries the tooth is displaced, usually as a result of fracture of the alveolar bone. The area needs to be anaesthetized, any fractures reduced, and the tooth splinted. Severely intruded teeth (>6mm in adults) usually required surgical repositioning and orthodontics. These patients require painkillers, antibiotics, and a mouthwash to keep the teeth clean as they are too tender to brush.

Avulsion

The tooth can be lost from its socket. This is much more common in children, as in adults the tooth is more likely to fracture. Advice can be given over the telephone to reimplant the tooth but you must always check the patient (even dentists have been known to replace the tooth the wrong way round). See p. 199 for the technique but make sure that the tooth is whole before reinserting it. It is advisable to place the tooth in milk while transferring to A&E.

Missing teeth

If you have just broken bad news about a lost tooth/crown, it is good to let patients know what options they have to close the gap.

- Crown—if there is enough root left in the socket a dentist can fabricate a crown which is retained by a post and core. This takes several appointments to make.
- Denture—can replace one or many teeth. It can be used temporarily to hold the space while a crown or implant is being made.
- Bridge—if the adjacent teeth are healthy they can be used to suspend a crown to cover the gap. Various types are available. Temporary bridges can again be used while a crown or implant is being prepared.
- Implant—these are expensive and not suitable for everyone. Although they can give an excellent result, the entire process can take months. They are not generally available on the NHS unless part of teaching/research.

Dento-alveolar infections

Overview

- Toothache without oro-facial complications is a dental problem and is not covered in this chapter.
- Pathogenesis: bacteria invade the pulpal chamber of the tooth leading to pulpitis, and then pulp necrosis. Infection spreads apically from root into bone and then soft tissues (Fig. 4.5), leading to sinusitis, cellulitis, or abscess. However, initial infection may be of the gum (periodontitis) or pericoronal tissues (pericoronitis).
- Dento-alveolar infections were the most common cause of death in under 20 year olds in the pre-antibiotic era.
- Cellulitis spreading through head and neck tissue planes (□ see p. 31) can lead to life-threatening oedema and airway obstruction, septi-caemia, cavernous sinus thrombosis, or tracking infection into the mediastinum.
- The majority of dento-alveolar infections are mixed anaerobic–aerobic infections and respond to broad-spectrum antibiotics, but pus should never be left undrained.

Assessment

Take a history of the toothache and associated symptoms. On examination, look for the following severity markers.

- **Airway compromise**—drooling. Very serious and possibly life threatening if you see this.
- **Raised floor of mouth (FOM)**—place gloved finger under tongue to examine.
- **Restricted tongue protrusion** can indicate a sublingual space infection.
- **'Hot potato voice'**—sublingual space infection or raised floor of mouth.
- **Pain on turning the head** may indicate a lateral pharyngeal space infection.
- **Trismus**—indicates possible submasseteric space infection.
- **Swelling**
- **Temperature** >38.5°C—'swinging pyrexia' with abscess.
- **Tachycardia**
- **Postural hypotension**
- **Raised white cell count**
- **Abscess**—collection of pus (inflammatory exudates, dead white cells). Fluctuant tense tender swelling which requires drainage and removal of source.

Causes of swelling

- **Oedema**—swelling of the tissues secondary to fluid retention. Common initial change in dento-alveolar infection in children

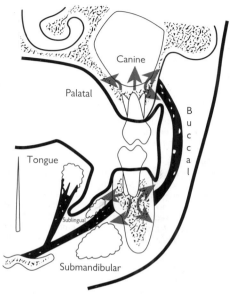

Fig. 4.5 Possible routes of spread of odontogenic infections. Reproduced from *Emergency Medicine Journal*, Antoun JS, Features of odontogenic infections in hospitalised and non-hospitalised settings, 2010 with permission from BMJ Publishing Group Ltd.

- **Cellulitis**—Intra- and inter-cellular oedema with rapid migration of bacteria though tissues—red, hot, and swollen tissue, often well demarcated on face. it can be treated with antibiotics and removal of cause.

Management

- Bloods including white cell count (WCC), C-reactive protein (CRP), glucose. Consider cultures.
- IV access and rehydrate.
- Commence IV broad-spectrum antibiotics, consider corticosteroids.
- OPG.
- Admit.
- Keep NBM.
- CT/US can sometimes be warranted—consult with senior. Sometimes collections can be drained under US guidance.
- If warranted, list for emergency theatre for incision and drainage under GA.
- Consent for intra-oral ± extra-oral drainage and extraction of teeth as necessary.

Antibiotics

Antibiotics can treat cellulitis effectively, but are not effective for abscesses. They are useful to help 'localize' abscesses, such that drainage is more straightforward, but beware trying to treat patients with anti-biotics alone—the offending tooth must be treated or extracted.

Drainage

Drain the pus! Infection causing pus formation associated with teeth is rarely treated successfully with antibiotics and analgesics alone. Oedema can also benefit from decompression.

• intra-oral drainage—incision in buccal mucosa.
• extra-oral drainage—incision through skin. Allows better drainage by gravity if the infection has tracked below the level of the jaw.

Ludwig's angina

This is a bilateral cellulitis affecting sublingual and submandibular spaces, such that the whole neck looks swollen. Often the FOM is raised and the tongue pushed up, restricting the airway. This is a life-threatening condition. Inform the registrar/consultant and get senior anaesthetic help to secure the airway. May require a fibre-optic intubation or a surgical airway (📖 see p. 208). Get IV access and arrange emergency decompression/ drainage as soon as possible. Commence IV antibiotics ± steroids in the meantime.

Periorbital cellulitis

Cellulitis generated by rapid migration of bacteria through the tissues around the eye. Often the source is the paranasal sinuses, but it can arise from the teeth, particularly the upper canines. Treat with IV antibiotics, incision, and drainage if pus has collected, and dental extraction if indicated.

Drains

Always obtain consent from patients undergoing incision and drainage for the possible placement of drains and sutures. Drains can be manufactured out of most things. The aim is to keep the abscess cavity open to the outside, allowing further exudates to drain.

• Possible materials:
  • Yates' drain (corrugated plastic)
  • rubber glove finger
  • ribbon gauze.
• Secure the drain with a silk suture,
• Pulling or 'shortening' the drain out in stages postoperatively allows the cavity to gradually close up behind it.

Post-extraction complications

Risks for complications include the following.

- *Patient factors* ♀ > ♂, elderly patient, African Caribbean, larger patient, smoking, medical problems (diabetes mellitus, Paget's disease, previous radiotherapy, bisphosphonates), poor oral hygiene (OH).
- *Tooth factors* Mandible > maxilla, third molars, unfavourable anatomy of tooth (e.g. divergent roots), hypercementosis, brittle tooth (e.g. large restoration), RCT.
- *Extraction factors* Single extraction, difficult extraction, bone removal, junior surgeon.

Bleeding (📖 see pp. 240 and 242)

Bleeding can be classified as follows.

- Primary haemorrhage—at time of extraction.
- Reactionary haemorrhage—up to 24 hours after extraction (usually after the vasoconstrictor has worn off).
- Secondary haemorrhage—more than 24 hours after extraction. Indicates infection.

Pain

Most patients will experience pain after extraction and simple analgesics are recommended. In difficult wisdom tooth extraction, especially those requiring bone removal, pain and swelling can be marked and usually peak at 4a.m. on the day after the surgery. It can be severe for 2–3 days; they will need time off work. Non-steroidal anti-inflammatory drugs (NSAIDs) often work best and can be used in combination with simple analgesics such as paracetamol.

Diagnosis

History

Onset of pain. Pain immediately after the LA has worn off suggests it is from a traumatic extraction or possibly fracture of adjacent tooth or bone. Dry socket pain typically starts after a few days.

Examination

Look for temperature, lymph nodes, halitosis, trismus, and the extent of any swelling. Fibrin in the clot becomes yellow from absorbing saliva so don't be fooled into thinking it is pus. If you can see bone, suspect dry socket or osteomyelitis.

Investigation

May need to X-ray the extraction site to show any retained fragments or fractures. Test adjacent teeth for sensitivity.

Causes of post-extraction pain
- Pain from extraction
- Dry socket
- Retained root or bone spicules
- Damage to adjacent tooth giving pulpal pain
- Dislocated mandible
- Haematoma
- Fractured bone
- Osteomyelitis (late)
- Osteonecrosis

Dry socket
Failure of retention of the clot within the socket because of vigorous rinsing or the action of lytic organisms (but *not* an infection). The incidence is much increased if the patient smokes, so avoid cigarettes for 24 hours after extraction. Contraceptive pill also increases risk. Severe throbbing pain ± lymphadenopathy typically onset 3–5 days after extraction. Grey–white bone is visible in the bottom of the socket (irrigate to have a look), hence its name *alveolar osteitis*. Treatment is irrigation with chlorhexidine, packing the socket with obtundant dressing such as Alvogyl®, analgesia, and review in a few days. Antibiotics are usually not indicated. This is a self-limiting condition, but very rarely spreading infection may develop. If it fails to heal suspect osteomyelitis or even malignancy—will need biopsy.

Swelling
This is normal after extraction. Trismus may be marked. Haematomas can rapidly form, but most can be left unless they are affecting the FOM or parapharyngeal regions. Once you have checked that there are no signs of infection or airway obstruction, the patient can be reassured. Some advocate ice packs.

Infection
This is rare, as the source of infection (tooth) has been extracted. Delayed swelling, bleeding, and pain are signs. Irrigate the socket, drain any collections, and prescribe antibiotics and hot salt-water mouth rinses. Osteomyelitis can develop, especially in immune compromise, so treat promptly.

Oro-antral communication
Roots of the upper molar teeth can extend into the maxillary sinus and when removed may leave a communication between the mouth and nose. Patients complain of fluid coming out of the nose when drinking or symptoms of sinusitis. Examine the extraction site and, if suspected, ask the patient to gently blow out of the nose. You may hear air coming out of the socket. This can be treated by a simple flap electively, but in A&E prescribe antibiotics and arrange follow-up. Packing with Surgicel® and a suture will do no harm. If left, a fistula will form which is more difficult to treat.

Dislocated mandible

There have been reports of patients being discharged after an extraction with a dislocation (□ see p. 200).

Parasthesia/anaesthesia

Nerves can be damaged by the LA injection as well as by the extraction itself. This is more common in the lower molar teeth. If there is still a feeling of numbness long after the LA has worn off, neuropraxia or even more permanent nerve damage (such as neurotmesis) is a possibility. If it was a difficult extraction, the patient should have been warned about this. Most cases resolve spontaneously, albeit slowly (up to 18 months). If there is any suggestion that the nerve was severed rather than crushed, referral for re-anastamosis is indicated.

Other common problems

- Suture falling out—if there is no bleeding, no treatment is needed.
- Retained root—most require extraction unless planned or too difficult to retrieve (i.e. close to nerve). Roots are sometimes left electively— the patient will have been told. Coronectomy has been advocated by some as an alternative to exodontia for third molars.
- Displaced fragment—parts of teeth can end up in many spaces in the head and neck. Arrange for follow-up to explore properly.
- Osteonecrosis—becoming more of a problem. Historically was seen in radiotherapy fields, but now bisphosphonate osteonecrosis can also occur. The mandible is more commonly affected than the maxilla. Seek senior help. In advanced cases, may need elective resection and re-construction.

Head and neck soft tissue infections

- Spreading infection from deeper structures such as teeth, sinuses, salivary glands, and bone is common and must be excluded.
- The surrounding anatomy can become involved, resulting in serious complications such as cavernous sinus thrombosis, airway obstruction, and even mediastinitis (common cause of death in medieval times!).

Localized infections

Carbuncle/furuncle/folliculitis

Staphylococcus aureus is the usual cause of infected hair follicles (folliculitis), most commonly in the beard area (sycosis vulgaris—'barber's itch') and scalp. Hot compresses and antibacterial skin wash may help mild cases; otherwise, systemic antibiotics are indicated. Take a pus sample to confirm the antibiotic choice (usually flucloxacillin). Furuncles and carbuncles are on a continuum of larger and deeper infected nodules and usually require incision and drainage. Look for a precipitating cause (e.g undiagnosed diabetes) random blood glucose is useful as initial test.

Impetigo

Superficial staphylococcal/streptococcal infection causing golden-crusted pustular lesions. It is common in children and often presents on the face. The sores are highly contagious and very itchy, so meticulous hand hygiene is required. Families should not share towels and bedclothes. Topical fusidic acid ± oral flucloxacillin is usually effective.

Infected/inflamed epidermoid (sebaceous) cyst

Cysts originating from the sebaceous glands are commonly found on the face and scalp. Infected cysts are acutely painful until spontaneous bursting or incision relieves the pressure. The cyst can be incised in A&E with ethyl chloride spray to anaesthetize. Wait until the skin suddenly goes white and then incise quickly before sensation is regained (LA is very unlikely to work). A finger from a sterile rubber glove can be secured with a nylon suture or a Penrose drain inserted into the cavity to prevent the cyst from re-forming. Follow-up is required for formal excision of the cyst once infection has cleared (📖 see p. 144).

Chronic draining sinus

Chronic periapical infection can lead to pus tracking through alveolar bone and out onto the skin, classically a spot under the chin draining from the lower incisor teeth. There may be no oral pain unless the draining sinus becomes blocked. The skin infection will not respond to topical or systemic antibiotics; the offending tooth needs to be extracted.

Spreading infection

Erysipelas

A bright red painful spreading infection of skin which is raised, firm, and hot to touch. It is usually due to inoculation of a minor wound (e.g. insect bite) with endogenous Group A *Streptococcus* from the nasopharynx. The rash quickly spreads and can progress to blistering and necrosis if severe. Blood cultures are indicated if the patient has a high temperature, and penicillin remains first-line therapy.

Necrotizing fasciitis

This thankfully rare condition has a high mortality, particularly when involving the cranio-cervical region. The infection is usually polymicrobial, including both aerobic and anaerobic organisms. There is rapid spread along the deep fascial planes and necrosis of the subcutaneous tissues. Prompt surgical debridement and broad-spectrum intravenous (IV) antibiotics (discuss with microbiology as flora will differ between patients (e.g. IV drug users) are the mainstay of treatment. Hyperbaric oxygen has been shown to reduce mortality but is not widely available. Overwhelming sepsis is common, and most patients will be treated on ITU. Spread to the mediastinum is invariably fatal.

Cellulitis

Facial cellulitis can develop from infection introduced through a break in the skin (e.g. after a punch to the face) or from infection of deep structures—the so-called 'fat face' associated with dental infections. The source of infection must be addressed to control the cellulitis. The most serious form of this is ▶▶ *Ludwig's angina*, where spreading cellulitis in the floor of the mouth can lead to airway obstruction. Patients are often very septic and require urgent anaesthetic involvement to secure the airway followed by surgical drainage of the infection. Always feel under the tongue to assess for swelling in the FOM (📖 see p. 233).

Periorbital cellulitis

Cellulitis can develop around the eye following infection of the upper teeth or, more commonly, sinusitis. It is critical to differentiate between pre- and post-septal cellulitis. Pre-septal cellulitis is infection limited posteriorly by the orbital septum. Patients have swollen eyelids but no ocular pain or restriction in eye movement. This can sometimes be managed by oral, rather than IV, antibiotics. Orbital (post-septal) cellulitis is a surgical emergency. Patients have proptosis, ophthalmoplegia, and diplopia. IV antibiotics are always required to prevent complications such as meningitis, brain abscess, and cavernous sinus thrombosis. Urgent CT is indicated, and definitive treatment is usually managed by ENT colleagues who can endoscopically drain the infected paranasal sinuses.

Viral infections

Shingles

Herpes zoster infection—reactivation of the varicella (chickenpox) virus—causes severe pain in a dermatome together with vesicles/blistering. The trigeminal nerve is commonly involved in the head and neck. Infection of the ophthalmic division can result in blistering and subsequent scarring of the cornea, so urgent ophthalmic referral and antiviral therapy is indicated. Post-herpetic neuralgia is severe and more common in the older age group. Zoster normally affects the sensory nerves. The notable exception to this is *Ramsay Hunt syndrome* where infection of the geniculate ganglion causes paralysis of the facial nerve (look for telltale vesicles in the external auditory meatus and fauces—the facial nerve has sensory branches to these areas!) Liaise with the medical team about ongoing management.

Salivary gland diseases

- In the emergency setting most gland problems will be related to infection or obstruction, but you must consider the possibility of a salivary neoplasm or underlying connective tissue disorder. Always review patients once the acute problem has settled.
- Painless discrete swellings with associated lymphadenopathy and nerve palsy are red flag signs (and suggest malignancy).
- Be extremely careful when suturing mucosa around the salivary ducts. You can inadvertently obstruct them (📖 see pp. 12, 26). Papillotomy can be performed for stones visible at the duct opening. Inject a small amount of LA and open the papilla with a No.11 blade. The stone should pop out with a gush of saliva. Leave the incision open and advise chewing gum and hot salt-water mouth rinses in the healing period.
- Description is based on old terminology—'sialaden' for salivary gland. Hence inflammation is sialadenitis, atrophy is sialectasis, contrast investigation is a sialogram, and stones are sialolithiasis.

Infection

Bacterial

Acute bacterial sialadenitis is an extremely painful infection usually of the parotid or occasionally the submandibular gland. The affected gland is tenderly swollen and erythematous, and the patient (typically a de-hydrated elderly patient, often with poor oral hygiene) may be quite unwell. Pus can be expressed from the duct (swab it and send for microbiology). *S.aureus* is the usual organism. Prompt IV co-amoxiclav and IV fluids are required. US scan may reveal an abscess requiring surgical drainage. Chronic infection may necessitate gland excision (📖 see p. 166).

Viral

Mumps (paramyxovirus) is relatively rare since widespread vaccination, but should be suspected in any acute swelling of the major salivary glands. The swelling is not always bilateral and can affect other organs such as the pancreas and testes (71% infertility). There is a classical mumps voice, and patients complain of arthralgia, lethargy, and headache. Treatment is symptomatic. Mumps is a notifiable disease in the UK, so serum samples for IgG and IgM as well as buccal swabs for mumps virus should be taken.

Viral sialadenitis can also be caused by HIV, cytomegalovirus (CMV), Epstein–Barr virus (EBV), and para-influenza virus.

Obstruction

Salivary gland stones

These are most commonly found in the submandibular gland where blockage of Wharton's duct causes repeated painful swelling of the gland when salivation is induced—'meal-time syndrome'. Bimanual palpation of the gland may reveal the presence of a stone, which can be removed if it is at the papilla. The high calcium content of the stones means that 70% are visible on plain X-ray (e.g. lower standard occlusal for submandibular gland stones). Conversely, US scans are not good at showing stones unless they are within the gland. Ascending bacterial infection can result from obstruction and requires admission if severe. However, these patients are usually best managed in the outpatient setting.

Mucocoeles and mucous retention cysts

Minor salivary glands in the labial mucosa and FOM can become damaged by minor trauma, resulting in swelling and cyst formation. When found under the tongue these are called 'ranula'. Although not very painful, they can be worrying when they appear suddenly and prompt a visit to the emergency department. The patient can be reassured and excision of the cyst plus gland arranged for an elective locals list. If they are very large, they can be decompressed with a needle as a temporary measure.

Trauma

The superficial position of the parotid gland means that it can be relatively easily injured. One particularly charming wound inflicted on informers, 'the telephone', involves slashing the side of the face with resultant parotid and facial nerve damage. The sublingual and sub-mandibular glands are relatively well protected by the mandible.

- Examine for nerve injury before administering local anaesthetic.
  All nerve injuries require formal exploration in theatre.
- Disrupted ducts need re-anastamosis and stent insertion in theatre.
  A plastic cannula sheath inserted into the duct intra-orally can
  demonstrate a transected duct when it appears in the wound.
- Careful closure of the parotid fascia can prevent a salivary fistula.
- Most salivary fistulae will resolve spontaneously with pressure
  dressings.

Miscellaneous conditions

Facial nerve palsy

The causes are legion but diagnosis is idiopathic (i.e. Bell's palsy) in ~75% of cases. Don't forget that this is a diagnosis of exclusion. Check whether the lesion is upper (forehead sparing) or lower motor neuron, unilateral or bilateral. Check the muscles of facial expression, test for hyperacusis (pain on loud noise because of absent stapedius reflex), corneal reflex, taste, and salivary flow, and examine ears and pharynx for viral lesions. Complete neurological examination is indicated.

Causes of CN VII palsy

This is not an exhaustive list
- Vascular—stroke.
- Tumour—CN VII can be compressed anywhere along its length, e.g intracranial (cerebello-pontine angle, acoustic neuromas), cranial base and, parotid tumours.
- Trauma—cranial base fracture, facial laceration.
- Infective—herpesviruses most commonly, e.g Ramsay Hunt syndrome (herpes zoster—look for vesicles in the ear). Others include Guillain–Barré syndrome (may be bilateral) and Lyme disease.
- Neurological—multiple sclerosis and other degenerative conditions, e.g amyotrophic lateral sclerosis.
- Infiltrative—sarcoid, leukaemia.
- Bell's palsy—can be considered if the above are excluded. Unilateral lower motor neuron lesion in an otherwise well patient. Possibly a viral trigger and is usually self-limiting.
- Rare syndromes, e.g Heerfordt's syndrome—uveitis, fever, parotid swelling.
- Iatrogenic—damage due to surgery.

Management
- Exclude serious cause—CT or MRI may be indicated.
- Protect the eye—warn the patient, eye drops, patch (not long term).
- Studies have shown that prescription of 50mg prednisolone daily for 10 weeks can reduce the time to recovery if commenced within 24 hours of onset of symptoms. The use of aciclovir is more controversial, but is certainly indicated if there is evidence of viral infection.

Bleeding gums

The most common cause of bleeding gums is gingivitis, 'gum disease'. Bleeding occurs when the gums are touched and is usually noticed by the patient when they spit out blood-stained toothpaste. Improving oral hygiene will improve gingivitis.

Spontaneous bleeding of the gums may reflect a more serious condition such as:

- acute necrotizing ulcerative gingivitis (ANUG), also known as 'trench mouth' as described in the frontline soldiers in the First World War. A combination of poor oral hygiene, stress (or any cause of immune suppression), and smoking can predispose to infection by multiple anaerobes, giving symptoms of painful necrotic bleeding gums, halitosis, lymphadenopathy, and fever. Treatment is oral metronidazole and chlorhexidine mouthwash, although the condition can resolve without treatment. Oral hygiene must be reviewed once the acute symptoms have settled, together with smoking cessation and investigation of immune suppression (e.g HIV).

- Clotting disorder—inherited or acquired. Check medications and alcohol use, and perform clotting screen.
- Leukaemia—classically, acute myeloid leukaemia (AML) causes sudden gingival enlargement (infiltration with leukaemic cells) with bleeding (↓platelets). A blood film should reveal the diagnosis. Severe gingival bleeding can be tamponaded by taking a conventional impression.

Pericoronitis

The gum overlying a partially erupted lower wisdom tooth is prone to painful inflammation due to:

- trauma from opposing upper wisdom tooth;
- infection from organisms trapped under the gum flap, an ideal breeding ground for anaerobes.

Spreading infection is rare but there can be severe pain, swelling, trismus, and lymphadenopathy.

Management

- Irrigate under the operculum (gum flap) using a Monoject syringe (has a curved tapered nozzle) filled with chlorhexidine mouthwash. Show the patient how to do it so they can continue at home.
- Analgesia.
- If there is spreading infection, prescribe antibiotics (IV if very severe).
- Refer for extraction if there have been >2 episodes (NICE guidelines) or if severe.
- In the acute situation extraction of the opposing tooth may relieve pain.

Earring tear

The lower pole of the ear lobe can be completely torn through, resulting in an unsightly forking of the lobe. If the injury presents immediately, repair is simple with direct closure of the skin on both surfaces of the lobe. Unfortunately, if patients present more than a few days after the injury, the surfaces will be epithelialized and simple suture will not be possible. The scar tissue must be removed and the bleeding surfaces opposed. However, in these days of funding cuts it is a treatment that may not be available on the NHS.

In the clinic

OMFS clinics

These include outpatient clinics, pre-admission clinics, and minor surgery/local anaesthetic clinics. OMFS clinics are often a mixture of all of these, so you have to be adaptable and so do the nurses. For example, you may be doing an outpatient clinic and be asked to perform an urgent biopsy of a suspected cancer or remove an upper wisdom tooth which is traumatizing the operculum of its counterpart.

The nurses
- Many of the nurses will be dental nurses.
- Dental nurses are skilled at assisting you, mixing materials (e.g. for impressions), and disinfection policies. They are also very good at calming anxious patients.
- They have also probably been there longer than you and will still be there after you have gone.
- However, it will be you in front of the General Medical Council, not them, so don't do anything you are not happy with and be confident in what you know.
- You would be unwise to attempt any procedures/examinations without having someone else in the room with you.

Minor surgery
- If you think you need help with a procedure talk to a supervisor before you start. Make the most of having a senior around; it will be invaluable learning for when you are on call on your own.
- Make sure that you adequately consent the patient. Most hospitals require written consent even for LA procedures.
- Sharps injuries are much too common. Clear away your own sharps; then everyone knows whose responsibility it is.
- See sections on anaesthesia and suturing techniques (📖 see pp. 190, 193).

Equipment
- You will often find that the consulting room has a dental chair.
- You may not have to use it for consultation but you will usually need it for examination and any clinical procedures. Familiarize yourself with the controls early as it can be embarrassing otherwise.
- Many patients require radiographs. Radiographs may be obtained by dentists or dental nurses with appropriate training in the clinic (📖 see p. 4 regarding legal requirements to take your own radiographs). Otherwise send radiology requests early to avoid delays in the clinic.

Pre-admission clinics

- The general clerking is the same as for any operation and the same rules apply. Examine the whole patient, ensuring that you have all the necessary results, and if you request any tests it is your responsibility to obtain the results prior to the operation.
- In maxillofacial surgery, we are sharing the airway with the anaesthetist so at the pre-assessment clinic you must consider what sort of airway will be required. Will it be an oral or nasal endotracheal tube? Will a tracheostomy be required? Will it be done at the start or the end of the procedure? Will the pathology make the intubation difficult? If you have any doubts, contact the anaesthetist at this stage. If the intubation is likely to be difficult, the anaesthetist will usually want to see the patient themselves well before the operation. They may need endoscopes and extra help.
- You should be familiar with a procedure before obtaining consent. Don't forget to warn the patient about drains, dressings, and restrictions such as elastics that they will have to contend with after the operation.
- Each unit should have a policy on preoperative bloods. Always check whether you need to group and save or cross-match blood, and send off a sickle screen if indicated. Not doing this can delay lists and will not make you popular.

Mandible fractures

Patients whom you see in the clinic will be there either for a postoperative review (e.g. 2 and 6 weeks post-surgery) or for fractures that are being managed conservatively, who may possibly need surgery.

Plates used for fixation are left *in situ* unless they are causing symptoms or in children.

Postoperative review

History
- What did they have done/when? Where are the plates? (Confirm with operation note and pre/postoperative films).
- Swelling should be improving by 2 weeks post-surgery.
- Difficulty in eating—weight loss is not uncommon.
- Feeling of malocclusion—is it getting worse or better?
- Numbness.

Examination
- Remove elastics and assess mouth opening.
- Note oral hygiene, and assess occlusion plus wound healing. Is there a plate exposed?
- Any fracture site mobility? ❶Call senior.
- Record any numbness diagrammatically.
- Painful teeth—teeth may have become non-vital due to trauma and periapical infection can develop.
- Radiographs are not usually indicated unless there is a problem.

Problems
- Occlusion not correct—always discuss this with a senior. Intermaxillary fixation (IMF) intervention may be possible before resorting to further surgery (teeth can move!). Options depend on when the surgery was done and the complexity of the fracture.
- Poor OH—the patient may assume that they shouldn't brush their teeth, so reinforce that they should and that mouthwash alone is not enough. Consider whether IMF can be removed to aid cleansing.
- Poor wound healing/breakdown—Corsodyl® mouthwash and improved OH. Review.
- Loose IMF—tighten/take off. Patients will come to clinic to have the arch bars removed. This may be quite uncomfortable as the wires can become deeply embedded.
- Plate removal if pain/infection/palpable. This usually needs to be done in theatre.
- Trismus—patients should be encouraged to move the jaw early after surgery to prevent fibrous healing. Painless restriction in mouth opening can be improved by physiotherapy or a device such as a Therabite®. MUA is rarely indicated to break adhesions, but can be required especially after intra-capsular fractures.
- Paraesthesia—must check if this was present preoperatively. It can improve (can take up to 2 years) and they will get used to it. Discharge at 6 weeks if the fracture is OK and sensation is returning.

- Non-union—rare in the facial skeleton. Consider diagnosis of pathological fracture.
- Osteomyelitis—rare but consider.
- Children require special attention. Plates are routinely removed after 6 weeks as the bone overgrows. Growth disturbance and ankylosis can result from trauma, so any sign of asymmetry must be recorded and followed up.

Conservative management

Patients who have undisplaced/minimally displaced fractures can be managed conservatively and observed if they are comfortable.

- Weekly review is recommended for the first few weeks.
- Consider surgery if there is pain or increasing malocclusion.
- Check that they are they being compliant with a soft diet only.
- Radiographs are not routinely indicated unless there is a change in the clinical picture.

Orbital floor fractures

- The key to managing these patients well is making sure that you obtain a proper clinical review of the eye.
  - Orbit injuries must be seen by an ophthalmic surgeon.
  - If there is no obvious trauma to the globe but eye signs are present you need to obtain a full orthoptic assessment.
- In the clinic you will see:
  - patients in whom there is not a definite diagnosis yet;
  - patients with orbital floor fractures but no decision to operate has been made yet;
  - patients with orbital floor fractures who are being managed conservatively (but there is always small chance that they might need surgery);
  - postoperative patients.
- The decision to operate is complicated by trying to predict who will become symptomatic. Surgery is best performed within 2 weeks, but post-trauma swelling may initially mask diplopia and enophthalmos.

Diagnosis (📖 see p. 72)

Diagnosis is usually made on CT scan. Discuss treatment planning with a senior. Delayed surgery might require custom-made implants, which are expensive. Re-do's have a worse prognosis, so it is important to get it right first time.

- Indications for surgery.
  - Obvious enophthalmos.
  - Obvious hypoglobus.
  - Likely to develop enophthalmos (eye sunken in) or hypoglobus (eye pushed down), i.e. large defect/hammocking behind the axis of the orbit.
- Relative indications.
  - Diplopia may be an indication **but it** could be due to swelling or optic nerve injury. A full orthoptic and ophthalmic assessment is needed to differentiate between nerve injury and change of orbital volume.

If a decision is made to manage conservatively, the patient may be discharged on the proviso that they can return to the clinic should any symptoms develop.

Postoperative

- Review the wounds (normally 5–7 days postoperatively). You may need to remove a nylon continuous suture, although various incisions are possible, some of which are not sutured
- Assess the eye position. Does the patient feel that the eye appears normal? They are the best judge of this
- Check for diplopia and visual fields (NB. swelling will affect this).
- Check your local policy on follow-up and whether or not ophthalmology need to review

- Advise patients to perform eye exercises to practice maintaining fields of vision. Warn them that this might be a little painful at first
- Children always require follow-up from ophthalmology as they might need extra-ocular muscle surgery.

Problems

Scars in this region normally heal extremely well and can become invisible in the creases around the eye. Scar retraction can sometimes cause ectropion (eyelid is pulled outwards and tissues inside the eyelid may be visible) or entropion (the eyelid folds in on itself and the eyelashes can be extremely irritating to the eye).

- Ectropion normally settles by itself. The patient should regularly massage the tissues with a moisturizer or silicone gel.
- Entropion needs to be reviewed by a senior as it is more likely to need treatment (e.g. oculoplastics).
- Residual enophthalmos: if the eye position has not been adequately corrected by surgery, it is usual to wait for a few months for the swelling to resolve and the eye position to settle. Any further surgery will need detailed planning but success rates are not good.

Zygoma fractures

Preoperative

Fractures of the zygomatic complex can be difficult to assess in the immediate post-injury period. If there is no urgent indication for surgery it is reasonable to ask these patients back to clinic in 5–7 days for a full assessment. However, some units like to operate early, so check your local policy.

Reassessment

- Feel the ZF suture, supra- and infra-orbital rims, and zygomatic buttress (and hence assess mouth opening).
- From above and behind the patient check the level of the arches bilaterally. Is there any flattening? Look for enophthalmos by assessing the position of the globes—retract the upper lids manually and see if the levels of the pupils are equal. Objective measurement can be made with a Hertel exophthalmometer.
- From the front you may be able to detect flattening or hypoglobus and look for a down-sloping lateral palpebral fissure (lateral canthus).
- Record sensation of the first and second division of the trigeminal nerve.
- Check the occlusion—in young patients the maxilla can be flexed, giving a premature contact on that side.
- Check eye movements and record any diplopia. Measure visual acuity.

Investigations

- Plain facial views—these do not need repeating if done in A&E.
- CT scan if a complex fracture—ideally with coronal reformatting.
- Orthoptic assessment—Hess chart to map any ocular involvement accurately.
- Ophthalmology review—may not be needed if the eye is not involved (e.g. isolated arch fracture).

Indications for surgery:

- **Aesthetic** (most common)—the timing of surgery is controversial but most surgeons feel that they are better able to judge the results on the table if swelling has gone down. Others prefer to operate immediately when the fracture has not started to repair.
- **Functional** (e.g. restricted mouth opening or inferolateral orbital fractures which leave the globe vulnerable)—a numb cheek is not an indication for surgery as it cannot be reliably improved.

Postoperative

- In the first 24 hours there is a small risk (0.03%) of retrobulbar haemorrhage (see 📖 p. 242), so eye observations are essential.
- You must document the instructions for eye observations clearly in the patient's notes.
- Patients are normally reviewed at 2 weeks post-surgery.
- Check the operation note and post-fixation X-rays.
- Assess the wounds and see that the bone is still reduced.
- Examine for diplopia and numbness. Most numbness will improve over time, but if there is still residual numbness at 18 months it is unlikely to recover.
- If all is satisfactory, the patient can be discharged with a warning to avoid contact sports for 6 weeks. If they are planning on scuba diving they should tell the instructor as it can affect sinuses.
- Plates are left unless they are causing problems (e.g. plates at the ZF suture can be visible if elderly or thin tissues).

Maxillary fractures

These injuries are usually the result of significant trauma and so present in the hospital rather than the outpatient department. Occasionally, the diagnosis may have been missed. Your suspicions should be aroused when there are bilateral black eyes and a deranged occlusion without a mandible fracture.

Isolated Le Fort I fractures can be managed conservatively if the segment is relatively stable (some are incomplete fractures). This is the recommended management in elderly denture wearers. The denture should be left out for 6 weeks, and a new pair will need to be made once the fracture has healed.

Postoperative

- Normally reviewed weekly or fortnightly (ensure postoperative radiographs are done unless advised otherwise).
- Look at the pattern of injury and assess all affected areas (e.g. condyle fractures). Check the intra-oral wound and other facial wounds.
- The patient will probably have arch bars, which can be very uncomfortable. See if the wires can be trimmed/adjusted and advise orthodontic wax to cover the sharper parts.
- Elastic bands may be used to guide the occlusion. Take them off to assess the bite and then decide with a senior if they need to be replaced.
- OH is often bad, so spend some time showing the patient how best to clean their teeth.
- Ask specifically about CSF leak. If this is new or not improving, obtain a CT scan and discuss with neurology/ENT.
- Midline palatal factures require rigid arch bars to stop the teeth rotating inwards.
- Assess for sensory nerve function.

Removal of arch bars

These are normally taken off at 4–6 weeks. A specific appointment will need to be made as it can take up to 45 minutes.

- Local anaesthetic infiltration into the buccal sulcus near each of the tying wires should render the patient comfortable.
- Double glove and wear goggles (the patient must also have eye protection).
- Unwind a little of the wire with a heavy clip (anticlockwise) and cut one side. Pull the clip straight out at 90° to the tooth surface while supporting the jaw with your non-dominant hand. The wire should pull through easily.
- Wires should be collected in a pot of water (e.g. denture pot) and must be disposed of safely.

Nose, naso-ethmoidal, and frontal bone fractures

Nose

Preoperative

- If considering MUA you should be able to demonstrate septal/nasal bone deviation with cosmetic/functional component.
- Make sure that the injury is not likely to be repeated before fixing it (i.e. *retired* boxers!).

Postoperative (MUA)

- External splints are normally removed at 1 week. You may also need to remove septal splints (internal) after ~24 hours.
- If the result is unsatisfactory, a definitive rhinoplasty will be necessary (if the septum is also deviated, it will be a septorhinoplasty). This can be done primarily or as delayed procedure in ≥3 months.
- It can take 6–12 months for all the swelling to disappear, so the result may not be apparent until this period has elapsed.

Naso-ethmoidal fractures

Preoperative

- Diagnosis— see p. 76.
- Occasionally these can be managed conservatively, but effectively they are open fractures, even to the cranial contents, and should have close follow-up.
- Indications for surgery include significant telecanthus, CSF leak, or nasal deformity. Most surgeons will prescribe antibiotics for CSF leak—test clear fluid with BM sticks (same glucose levels as serum) or send it for β_2 transferrin if your Trust has the money!
- Early liaison with ophthalmologists is wise because of the risk of damage to the lacrimal apparatus and possible ocular motility problems.

Postoperative

- Measure intercanthal distance and assess the form of the nose in profile.
- Ask about lacrimal function.
- Remove stitches and check the position of plates.
- These are difficult fractures to fix satisfactorily and the patient may have to accept a slight change in appearance.

Frontal fractures

- The frontal bone is thick and tough, apart from the area containing the frontal sinus. The size and shape of the sinus is highly variable.
- Significantly displaced simple frontal bone fractures are rare and indicate significant impact. They usually result in massive underlying brain injury.
- Fractures involving the frontal sinus are much more common and the management depends upon if the anterior ± posterior walls are involved.
    - Isolated anterior wall—these can be managed conservatively if only minimally displaced. Grossly displaced fractures can give an unsightly ridge on the forehead, which is an indication for surgery.
    - Posterior wall—there is now direct communication between the frontal sinus and the anterior cranial fossa. Surgery is indicated because the lifetime risk of cerebral abscess and meningitis is of the order of 60–70%. The procedure undertaken is cranialization of the frontal sinus (see p. 160). Antibiotics are usually prescribed.

Postoperative

- If the patient had the bicoronal approach, take out scalp clips at 7–10 days.
- Check for CSF leak.
- Advise about wound care (e.g. massage scar).
- Posterior wall fractures may have a slightly longer follow-up period, but if surgery has been successful the patient's lifetime risk of meningitis will have been reduced to that of the normal population.

Face and scalp soft tissue injuries

- Follow-up is not required for most simple lacerations that are sutured in the ED.
- Patients being seen in clinic would generally have complicated lacerations where:
  - healing is expected to be compromised (e.g. skin loss or contaminated)
  - further reconstruction is needed
  - scar revision may be required at a later date
  - there are injuries associated with the wound.
- Scarring is a normal and essential part of wound healing, even if it has been sutured. It is important to educate and reassure patients regarding the normal clinical course of a healing wound so they know what to expect.

Recently treated lacerations

- Assess wound healing.
- Look for cellulitis—don't confuse with normal erythema.
- If wound infection or cellulitis is suspected, take a wound swab and prescribe an empirical antibiotic such as flucloxacillin.
- If in doubt consult microbiology regarding antibiotic choice.
- May need surgical debridement.
- Generally require cleaning and redressing only.

Normal clinical course of a scar

- 1–2 weeks following injury, the wound appears nicely healed with a thin red line
- Continues to thicken for 4–6 weeks as collagen is laid down.
- Can be itchy and tender during this proliferative phase.
- Collagen deposition and resorption occurs in equilibrium as the scar remodels.
- The scar gradually softens, becoming paler.
- After 12–18 months, the scar should be pale and asymptomatic.

Removal of sutures

If the patient is being followed up in clinic, it may be a good opportunity to remove the sutures to save the patient returning to the dressing clinic or seeing the GP nurse.

- Sutures can be removed as follows:
  - eyelid, 3–4 days
  - face, 5–6 days
  - scalp, 7–10 days
  - ears, 10 days
  - back/neck, 10–14 days.
- If Dermabond® (cyanoacrylate) has been used, ask the patient to apply white soft paraffin after 7 days and gently massage, which will help the glue come off. Discourage picking.

Assessing the final result

The optimal scar is a thin flat pale line in a relaxed skin tension line, which does not traverse or contract anatomical boundaries or structures.

Advise the patient to massage the final wound with a moisturizer or simple cream to break up the scar tissue and to wear sun protection factor.

- For lip lacerations, ensure the vermilion border has been re-aligned.
- For wounds around the eyes, check for ectropion (scar tissue pulling the lower lid down and outwards which may cause a watery or red eye).

Management of unsightly, hypertrophic, or keloid scars

History

Why is the scar unsightly? Is it uneven, stretched, sunken, hyper-pigmented, hypopigmented, raised, hypertrophic, keloid, or tattooed? Is it inflamed and symptomatic? Look at other scars on the body to assess for whether the patient scars poorly.

- Hypertrophic scars are thickened and raised, but remain within their orginal borders. Disordered collagen, high wound turnover, and vascularity. Usually regress spontaneously, and respond to treatment more than keloid scars
- Keloid scars are thickened, raised, and extend beyond the boundaries of the original wound. Build up of collagen, with greater wound turnover and increased vascularity. 5–15 times more common in black population.

Monitor

Allow an inflamed scar to mature over 1 year. Consider taking clinical photographs.

Treatment options

- Surgery may simply result in a worse scar, so start with conservative options.
- Pressure clips/facemask: >24mmHg 18–24hrs/day for 4–6 months.
- Silicone gel: apply for 12–14hr/day for 2–3 months.
- Silicone tape/patches:
- Intralesional steroid: triamcinolone 20mg/cm scar to a maximum of 120mg. Course of four injections every 4–6 weeks. Reduces collagen levels, inflammation, pruritus, and tenderness. Side effects include pain on injection, hypopigmentation, crystalline deposits, telangiectasia, and atrophy.
- Topical vitamin A (retinoic acid) inhibits fibroblasts and vitamin E reduces fibroblast number, 5-fluorouracil (5FU) inhibits cell division, penicillamine prevents collagen cross-linking, and colchicine increases collagenase activity.
- Laser—can reduce pigmentation and inflammation.
- Scar excision and re-suture, serial excision, scar re-alignment.
- Z-plasty, W-plasty.
- Adjunctive therapy, such as radiation, brachytherapy, or steroids, may be used with surgery.
- Coleman fat transfer or fillers can be used to restore volume.

Other soft tissue problems

Haematoma

● May require evacuation to aid healing. Cover with antibiotics.

Foreign bodies

● Imaging may help to identify. CBCT is the best imaging modality for this.
● May not be necessary to remove (e.g. shotgun injuries).
● Low velocity may be more likely to become infected.
● Depends on anatomy.

Abrasions

● Clean at early stage.
● May require scrubbing under LA/GA to remove any ingrained dirt or debris and prevent 'tattooing'.
● Dress with appropriate dressing for moist wound. If in doubt discuss with wound nurse

Dento-alveolar: impacted teeth

Definition of an impacted tooth

'Any tooth that is prevented from reaching its normal position in the mouth by bone, soft tissue or another tooth'.

Most commonly impacted teeth are 8s, 3s, 5s, and supernumaries. These patients will be referred to OMFS by GDPs or orthodontists for assessment in clinic.

Impacted third molars

History

Pain history, number of episodes of pericoronitis and how severe—whether or not antibiotics required. Exclude other causes such as temporomandibular joint dysfunction syndrome (TMJDS). Relevant medical, dental, and social history. Assessment of anxiety.

Examination

- Extra-oral—facial swelling or asymmetry, lymphadenopathy, TMJ
- Intra-oral—inter-incisal opening, condition of rest of dentition, OH, position of lower third molars, position of upper third molars, position of external oblique ridge, condition of lower second molars, presence of pericoronitis, other features that may be of significance (removable prostheses, profound gag reflex, etc.).

Investigation

Assess root morphology, degree of bone impaction, proximity to IDN, and associated disease (e.g. cysts, hypercementosis, TMJ problems).

- OPG—position, angulation, root morphology, degree of bone impaction, decay in 7, associated pathology, hypercementosis, proximity to IDN. Look for: loss of lines, shadow over apex (juxta-apical radio-lucency), deviation of canal.
- CBCT—focused 3D imaging of the jaw and a better representation of the relationship of the roots of the third molar to the IDN.

Management

As surgery has associated risks and mandibular impacted third molars are very common, the NICE guidelines[1] should be followed in most cases:

- unrestorable caries
- non-treatable pulpal and/or periapical pathology
- cellulitis
- abscess
- osteomyelitis
- internal/external resorption of tooth or adjacent tooth
- fracture of tooth
- disease of follicle including cyst/tumour
- tooth/teeth impeding surgery or reconstructive jaw surgery
- within field of tumour resection
- two or more episodes of pericoronitis
- one severe episode of pericoronitis

1 NICE Guideline 2000/003a. *Guidance on the Extraction of Wisdom Teeth.* Issued 27 March 2000 (available online at: http://www.nice.org).

Options

Leave, extract ± coronectomy if high risk to IDN.[2]

Potential complications of surgery

Swelling, bleeding, pain, trismus, nerve damage (lingual nerve or IDN), infection or dry socket, oro-antral communication, damage to other teeth or their restorations (often predictable from OPG), fractured mandible.

Impacted canines

History

Usually asymptomatic and picked up at routine examination by dentist. May be unerupted.

Examination

Look for retained canines, angulation of lateral incisor. Palpate whether the impacted canines are buccal or palatal.

Investigations

Radiographs, parallax technique (see p. 45). Cyst, root resorption.

Management

Extraction of deciduous canines (aged 10). Leave canine *in situ*, surgically remove, expose and bond, transplantation. Be guided by orthodontist.

Exposure of unerupted teeth

Main objective is to remove any bone or soft tissue that is preventing eruption of the tooth ± bonding of orthodontic appliance to align into arch.

Impacted second premolars

Lower 5s usually lingual, upper 5s normally palatal.

Management

Leave, expose, or extract.

2 Renton T, Hankins M, Sproate C, McGurk M (2005). *British Journal of Oral and Maxillofacial Surgery* **43**: 7–12.

Dento-alveolar: jaw pathologies

These patients will normally be referred with pain, swelling, or a radiological abnormality that has been picked up by the dentist.

History

Swollen face, numb lip, pain, trismus, time course of symptoms.

Examination

Swelling, numb lip/chin (red flag), buccal/lingual expansion, displaced teeth, lymphadenopathy.

Investigations

- OPG
- Discuss with senior—CT/CBCT/MRI scan, biopsy, etc.
- When viewing imaging of any 'lesion':
  - note site, size, shape, outline, radiodensity, effects on surrounding structures, single or multiple lesions;
  - determine whether normal anatomy, artefactual, or pathological.
- If pathological, determine whether:
  - dental abnormality
  - bone abnormality
  - superimposed soft tissue calcification or salivary calculi.
  - foreign body.

Classification

- Cysts—odontogenic or non-odontogenic.
- Tumours—odontogenic or non-odontogenic, benign or neoplastic.
- Bone disorders—non-neoplastic or neoplastic.

Ten causes of multilocular radiolucency (Fig. 5.1)

- Keratocystic odontogenic tumour (odontogenic keratocyst)
- Ameloblastoma
- Ameloblastic fibroma
- Odontogenic myxoma
- Calcifying epithelial odontogenic tumour (CEOT or Pindborg tumour)
- Central giant cell lesion
- Brown tumour of hyperpara-thyroidism
- Cherubism
- Aneurysmal bone cyst
- Central haemangioma

Ten causes of a variable radiodensity lesion (Fig. 5.2)

- Calcifying epithelial odontogenic tumour (CEOT or Pindborg tumour)
- Ameloblastic fibro-odontoma
- Adenomatoid odontogenic tumour (AOT)
- Cementoblastoma
- Osteoma
- Osteogenic osteosarcoma
- Osseous dysplasia
- Familial gigantiform cementoma
- Fibrous dyplasia
- Ossifying fibroma

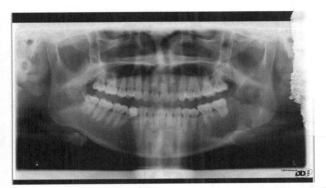

Fig. 5.1 Large multilocular expansile radiolucency, left posterior mandible (ameloblastoma).

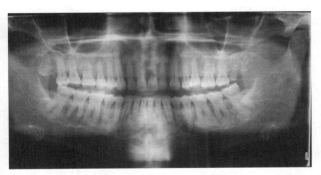

Fig. 5.2 Variable radiodensity lesion, bilateral mandible (fibro-osseous dysplasia).

Temporomandibular joint problems

- These patients can often be a challenge to diagnose accurately or treat effectively.
- The history and examination yields the vast majority of the information leading to accurate diagnosis.

TMJ anatomy

- The condylar head articulates with the glenoid fossa of the temporal bone.
- The TMJ is a synovial joint with a fibrocartilaginous disc.
- Ligaments include the temporomandibular ligament laterally, and the stylomandibular and sphenomandibular ligaments running medial to the joint.
- Muscles of mastication and their movements:
- Elevators: temporalis, masseter, medial pterygoid
- Protrusion: lateral and medial pterygoids
- Depression: lateral pterygoid, infra- and supra-hyoid muscles
- Lateral excursion: contralateral pterygoids and ipsilateral temporalis.

TMJ conditions

- TMJ dysfunction syndrome (TMJDS)
- Facial arthromyalgia or myofascial pain
- Ankylosis
- Trauma—condylar fracture, intracapsular fracture, effusion, dislocation
- Condylar hypo/hyperplasia
- Arthritides—degenerative or inflammatory
- TMJ neoplasia—benign or malignant (metastasis is also possible).

History

The features to ask about are pain, clicking, locking, trismus, history of trauma, other symptoms such as headache.

Examination

The features to examine for are joint tenderness or muscle of mastication tenderness, clicking on opening or closing, abnormal path of opening, evidence of parafunction (tooth wear), masseteric hypertrophy, bitten fingernails, scalloped tongue. Lower back pain, menorrhagia, headaches, IBS, pelvic pain—associated with TMJDS.

Investigations

- OPG (must include condylar heads)—asymmetry, flattening of condylar head.
- MRI scan—internal derangement.
- CT scan—condylar resorption, bony tumour.
- Computer-aided design/computer-aided manufacturing (CAD/CAM) or stereolithographic modelling.
- Study models for resorption (e.g. condylar resorption post orthognathic surgery).

Management

- A patient with painless click can be treated conservatively.
- Pain without a click (myalgia)—treat conservatively
- Pain with a click—internal derangement ± myalgia
- Is it reducible or irreducible (locking or not)?

Conservative

- Reassurance and education.
- Straight-line jaw exercises.
- Simple analgesia.
- Heat.
- Rest/soft diet/relaxation/modifying lifestyle.
- Splints/bite guards/bite-raising appliances—Michigan splint (upper) and Tanner splint (lower) work by opening up the joint space to free the disc, or possible placebo affect.
- If the splint abolishes the pain after 3 months and the pain returns when the splint is not worn, occlusal reorganization could be considered by restorative treatment—crowns or orthodontics.

Intervention

Consider anaesthetic implications—may require an awake fibreoptic or elective tracheostomy under LA if profound trismus.

Procedures

- Arthroscopy.
- Arthrocentesis—joint washout. Sometimes morphine is also placed in the joint with or without arthroscopy.
- Discectomy/menisectomy.
- Condylar shave.
- Eminectomy.
- Joint replacement—reserved for severe symptomatic endstage joint disease, adult ankylosis, neoplastic processes, or avascular necrosis. Done in specialist centres only.

Oral and facial pain

- Imagine the number of different structures in the head and neck region and you will appreciate that there are many possible causes for oral and facial pain.
- The key to diagnosis is in the history. In many patients the examination findings will not be helpful so listen carefully.

Toothache and TMJ disorders are discussed elsewhere in this book but below is a list of the more common pain conditions and their salient features:

Trigeminal neuralgia

- ♀ > ♂; unusual before the age of 50.
- Intense sharp shooting pain 'electric shock' in the distribution of CN V (unilateral and usually the maxillary or mandibular branch).
- Pain comes in pulsating spasms of seconds/minutes and is described as excruciating (severe enough for some patients to resort to suicide).
- There may be a specific trigger point which will result in the pain when touched (e.g. the patient avoids shaving a particular patch on cheek).
- No sensory or motor impairment, and examination is normal.

Causes

- Idiopathic.
- Diabetes—causes demyelination, check fasting glucose.
- Multiple sclerosis—look for other lesions (bladder, optic, etc.) and sensory or motor symptoms.
- Intracranial vascular compression of the trigeminal nerve—thought to be responsible for the pulsatile nature of the pain and the basis for treatment by microvascular decompression.

Space-occupying lesion

Check for other neurological signs, e.g. loss of corneal reflex found in cerebellopontine angle tumours.

Investigations

MRI/CT may be indicated to exclude a space-occupying lesion in brain, brainstem, or infra-temporal fossa, and is clearly essential if neurosurgical intervention is being considered for vascular decompresion.

Treatment

Long-lasting LA injection to infra-orbital nerve can be diagnostic and a short-term treatment. Carbamazepine is first-line treatment—dose is titrated to response but the effect can wear off after some years. Pheno/cryo-ablation of the nerve can be indicated and microvascular decompression to separate the geniculate ganglion from the intracranial vessels is effective evidence-based treatment (but 0.5% risk of death).

Other drugs used include gabapentin, baclofen and clonazepam.

Glossopharnygeal neuralgia

This is the same problem as trigeminal neuralgia but in a different distribution. Pain is in the unilateral base of tongue and can be triggered by swallowing, chewing, and coughing. Carbemazepine is effective.

Temporal arteritis

Typically >50 years of age. Pain in the temporal region and cheek, especially on chewing (masseteric claudication). Prompt treatment with IV steroid is required to prevent ocular sequelae. There may be a tender swollen non-pulsatile superficial temporal artery. Diagnosis is confirmed by biopsy of the artery (at least 2cm should be excised), but treatment may be instituted from examination findings and high ESR where biopsy cannot be arranged urgently.

Cluster headache (SUNCT, periodic migrainous headache)

Nine times more common in ♂; age group 30–50 years. Complain of recurrent headache, which usually occurs at the same time of day and can waken the patient—'alarm clock headache'. Usually unilateral and causes intense stabbing pain in distribution of V2 with reddening and tearing of the eye. Alcohol can be a precipitant. Prophylactic ergotamine or intranasal lidocaine can be effective.

Atypical facial pain and atypical odontalgia

Often there is a protracted history (many years) with multiple extractions of healthy teeth before this diagnosis is considered. Pain is often described as drawing or gripping and does not relate to normal anatomical boundaries. Although described as severe, the pain does not wake the patient from sleep or affect their diet. There may also be delusional symptoms such as powder coming out of the gums, or bizarre tastes such as oil or fish. The trick is to recognize this condition before rendering the patient edentulous. Counselling, cognitive behavioural therapy (CBT), and low-dose antidepressants have all be used as treatment (with varying success). Patients need to be informed that these conditions will not always be curable.

Burning mouth syndrome and oral dysaesthesias

More common in middle-aged females, especially peri-menopausal, which has led to suggestion of a hormonal cause. There is a burning sensation in the tongue and sometimes the whole mouth. Taste may be altered and some patients describe a feeling that the cheek mucosa peeling off and bad breath. Examination is entirely normal. Occasionally a cause can be found such as low iron or vitamin B_{12} levels (so always take bloods) and gastro-oesophageal reflux disease (symptoms worse in the morning and nasendoscopy shows oedematous vocal chords). Often a history of severe stress or depression can be found on probing, although the similarity of symptoms in these patients leads to an interesting discussion of the psychological versus the physical. Treatments such as CBT and nortriptyline have been shown to be effective. Some patients with normal bloods still improve with B_{12} supplements.

Management of oral lesions

- View the patient as a whole. Oral lesions are often manifestations of systemic disease, and this may be the first opportunity a clinician has to diagnose that condition.
- To biopsy or not to biopsy? Patients can be referred with oral ulcers, white patches, red patches, or mixed patches. Many of these will be benign, but this is impossible to confirm by clinical examination alone. Therefore histopathological diagnosis is required unless there is no doubt as to the benign nature of the lesion.
- 📖 See p. 211 for a more detailed description of the various conditions you are likely to see.

History

- How long has the lesion been present? Was it initially noticed by the patient or the dentist? Is it symptomatic and are there any other associated problems—otalgia, dysphagia, loose teeth?
- A detailed medical history, drug history, and social and family history are of great relevance. Look for risk factors such as smoking, chewing betel nut, or drinking alcohol.
- Do not neglect asking about genitourinary symptoms.
- ► **Warning signs**—non healing ulcers, pain or nerve involvement a late sign, history of alcohol, smoking, betel nut, human papilloma virus (HPV) infection.

Examination

- Examine outside the mouth first (scalp, face, and neck), particularly for lymphadenopathy.
- Intra-orally, examine all soft and hard issues in the mouth after having removed any dentures present (📖 see p. 34).
- Describe the lesion: sessile, pedunculated, reticulate, homogenous, heterogenous, erosive, atrophic. Do the lesions wipe off? Note its size, size, shape, and effects on adjacent structures (or effects of adjacent structures on it).
- Depending on findings, a systemic examination may be required (e.g. other sites of lymphadenopathy such as axillae and groin, abdomen for hepato-splenomegaly, breast, etc.) Genitourinary examination may also be also indicated in certain circumstances.

Investigations

- Ulcers
  - Biopsy (mandatory if lesion >3 weeks).
  - Bloods—FBC, vitamin B_{12}, folate, serum ferritin. Consider B vitamins, zinc, and autoantibody immunology and HLA screening.
  - Swabs.
- Vesiculobullous disorders—direct and Indirect immunofluorescence.

Conditions of definite premalignant potential
- Leukoplakia
- Erythroplakia
- Erythro-leukoplakia
- Chronic hyperplastic candidiasis

Conditions associated with increased risk of malignant changes
- Lichen planus (particularly atrophic form)
- Submucous fibrosis
- Syphilitic glossitis
- Sideropenic dysphagia

Treatment

Ulcers
- Chlorhexidine mouthwash can decrease length of ulceration.
- Topical LA (although sensitization can be a problem).
- Topical corticosteroids—e.g. betametasone rinses.
- If severe, consider oral prednisolone in a reducing dose (possibly with gastric cover such as omeprazole).
- Triamcinolone injections for major aphthae (if biopsy negative for malignancy).

White patches
- Patient education regarding risk factors, especially stopping smoking.
- Photograph.
- Monitor in clinic if risk factors, high-risk histological appearance, or high-risk site (floor of mouth, posterior tongue).
- Excision/ablation if biopsy shows dysplasia.

Red patches
- Excision/ablation

Management of neck lumps

- New referrals should ideally be seen in a designated neck lump clinic with access to all the diagnostic methods described below.
- This should not prevent a patient with a neck lump from being seen as soon as possible.
- Normal lymph nodes are not normally palpable.
- Palpable lymph nodes in young people are usually reactive to infection.
- Palpable lymph nodes in old people are usually metastatic, e.g. aero-digestive small cell cancer, thyroid, or from below the clavicle (lung, breast or gastrointestinal (Virchow's node)).

History

- When and where first noticed?
- Painful?
- Any discomfort on swallowing?
- Increasing in size?

Examination

Extra-oral

- Site, size, shape, fluctuance, compressibility, mobility, fixed to related structures, overlying skin, tenderness on palpation, associated lymphadenopathy.
- Any movement with sticking tongue out or swallowing.

Intra-oral

- Assess the soft tissues, gingivae and dentition in detail. Soft tissues should include oropharyngeal tissues—base of tongue, tonsillar fossa, and uvula.
- Bimanually palpate the submandibular glands.

ENT

- Preferably, nasoendoscopy should be performed at first presentation for a neck lump without known cause.

Investigations

Bloods

FBC, ESR, TFT, LDH, ACE, EBV, CMV, HSV, HIV, toxoplasmosis, blood film.

FNA cytology

This should also preferably be performed at first presentation. Open biopsy is usually contraindicated as it can cause tumour seeding and local spread. FNAC is inconclusive in 30% of cases. A Trucut biopsy can be considered in this case. This can be taken under US or radiological guidance.

Ultrasound

US can determine node architecture, cystic nature, extent, relationship to salivary glands, shape (ovoid more likely to be reactive, rounded suggestive of malignancy), and size. Colour flow Doppler is also useful for assessing whether hilar blood flow is normal or haphazard (seen in malignant nodes).

CT/MRI

Both are good at assessing nodal status, although probably not much better than US for lymphadenopathy.

Examination under anaesthesia (EUA), panendoscopy, and biopsy

Essential for any suspicious tumour not easily visualized. Blind biopsies are often taken in the unknown primary tumour scenario—tongue base, post-nasal space, etc.

Differential diagnosis of a neck lump

Developmental

- Branchial cyst—rare, present in childhood or in early adulthood.

Infective

- Tuberculosis—cervical tuberculous lymphadenitis suggests post-primary or reactivation of previously quiescent infection. May be accompanying pulmonary or evidence of past tuberculosis on chest radiograph.
- Cat scratch disease—single markedly enlarged node. Exposure to cats or history of a primary skin infection at the site of a scratch.
- Toxoplasmosis—young adults, immunocompromised.
- Brucellosis.
- Glandular fever—young adults.
- HIV infection—causes generalized lymphadenopathy.

Inflammatory

- Sarcoidosis

Neoplastic

- Benign
  - Salivary gland neoplasm—pleomorphic adenoma, Warthin's tumour
  - Carotid body tumour (paraganglioma)—arises from the carotid body at the carotid bifurcation. Usually found at the anterior border of the sternocleidomastoid. Moves horizontally but not vertically due to attachment to carotid vessel. Pulsation, thrill, or bruit can be palpated or auscultated.
  - Soft tissue benign neoplasms.
- Malignant
  - Metastatic malignancy—cervical lymph node metastasis from a head and neck cancer. Most likely squamous cell carcinoma or adeno-carcinoma.
  - Low neck/supraclavicular fossa metastasis—always think about pathology below the clavicles (although some head and neck cancers can spread directly to the lower neck nodes).

Work-up for major head and neck oncoplastic surgery

- Patients suspected of having oral/oropharyngeal cancer will generally be referred to the OMFS clinic on an accelerated pathway. In the UK, this is within 2 weeks.
- A newly referred patient will be seen in clinic by the consultant who will have made a diagnosis based on the history, clinical features, and initial investigations. Further investigations are required to formally stage the tumour and then the patient will be seen at a multi-disciplinary team (MDT) meeting to decide on the optimum treatment plan.
- Work-up relates to ensuring that all necessary investigation and preparation for surgery has been completed and the results are available.

For major head and neck cancer surgery, there are generally two work-up stages:

For MDT
You may be asked to present a patient at the head and neck MDT meeting. **Ensure that the following information is available.**
- Patient's history and examination; medical, social, dental, and family history.
- Include details such as relevant risk factors—smoking, drinking, betel nut use, patient comorbidity, medications, exercise tolerance, their ASA grade, and anything else that you think may affect which treatment they have.
- Imaging (OPG, CXR, CT scan) of head, neck, thorax, and upper abdomen for staging. Ensure appropriate re-formatting of scans are available, e.g. coronal views of paranasal sinuses.
- Have radiological reports (although a head and neck radiologist should be present at the MDT meeting).
- Further tests—MRI, CT-PET, US scans ± FNAC.
- Biopsy result and histopathological report.
- Ensure that it is known whether the patient has been informed of the diagnosis yet.

For surgery
Have the above ready, plus the following.
- Clear treatment plan agreed at MDT, including any adjunctive radio- or chemotherapy.
- Further reconstruction-based imaging.
- Dental assessment—patients must be dentally fit, or have a plan to have any teeth of poor prognosis extracted before treatment, as they may be having radiotherapy and at risk of developing osteoradio-necrosis.
- Bloods—have results available, including any requested by the anaesthetist on the morning of surgery. These include preoperative Hb, electrolytes, LFTs, and albumin.

- G&S and crossmatch—4 units for composite flaps, 2 units for soft tissue flaps and/or neck dissection (check local transfusion protocols).
- Nutrition
  - Know what the nutritional plan for the patient is postoperative
  - Enteral feeding—NGT or PEG/RIG
  - Parenteral feeding—rarely required in head and neck cancer patients
  - Ensure that dieticians and speech and language therapy (SALT) are aware of the patient
- Book an ITU bed—if not done, can result in the operation being postponed.

Specific reconstruction investigations

Radial flap

- Non-dominant forearm, check no previous surgery or Raynaud's syndrome, vascular investigations (Allen's test ± duplex US scan) to ensure patency of radial and ulnar arteries and the palmar arch.

Fibula flap

- Duplex US scan, conventional angiography, MR angiogram or CT angiogram (both are less invasive) to ensure that all three vessels in the leg are patent and healthy.

Deep circumflex iliac artery (DCIA) flap

- Ensure that there is no previous abdominal surgery, check medical/surgical history, and examine for scars.
- Scapular flap—no previous injuries or surgery.

Anterolateral thigh (ALT) flap

- Hand-held Doppler available for mapping the perforators pre-operatively.

Reviewing head and neck cancer patients

- The postoperative care of a head and neck cancer patient is centred on rehabilitation
- There are specific aspects of rehabilitation to focus on in the clinic to ensure that the clinic visit is worthwhile
- Good documentation of examination findings and any discussion with the patient or their carer is important
- Make use of specialist nurses and members of the MDT
- Regular assessment is required to ensure that treatment benefits are not outweighed by their side effects.

Assessing for postoperative recurrence

- Look carefully at the site of tumour, examine the neck bilaterally, check the flap donor site, and examine the PEG site.
- Further investigation for recurrence may include plain film radiographs, US scan, CT, or CT-PET. Endoscopic examination and biopsy may be required.

Assessing postoperative function

An 11-domain clinical examination was devised in Liverpool to assess the main postoperative functional deficits.[1] This is a useful examination to perform postoperatively to assess motor and sensory nerve function and to gauge the success of the reconstruction. The examination assesses:

- lip competence
- tongue movement
- oral mucosa
- dental state
- mouth opening
- speech
- drooling
- diet
- appearance
- oral sensation
- shoulder movement.

Assessments of speech and swallowing can be made clinically with the help of SALT. Special tests such as videofluoroscopy and fibreoptic endoscopic examination may also be required.

Assess OH and dental health, which are particularly at risk if the patient has had radiotherapy or sugar-laden fortified drinks, such as Ensure. Prosthetic rehabilitation will need to be planned with the help of restorative/prosthodontic dentists and technicians.

---

1 Rogers SN, Lowe D, Fisher SE, Brown JS, Vaughan ED (2002). *British Journal of Oral and Maxillofacial Surgery* **40**: 11–18.

Assessing quality of life

Various quality of life (QoL) indices are available which can be used to gain an overall understanding of how the patient's symptoms, function and pyschology are affected. These include the University of Washington (UoW) index, the EORTC questionnaire, and the Functional Assessment of Cancer therapy scale. These are all suitable for collecting comparative data on outcome after surgery.

There is no ideal questionnaire, and often the best approach is to listen to patients' direct concerns in the clinic, as they will have prioritized the issues themselves.

Note that QoL generally decreases for the first 3 months following major surgery. Postoperative QoL at 1 year is more indicative of the long-term outcome.

Assessing radiotherapy patients

- Short-term problems:
  - mucositis, loss of taste, dry mouth, infection, lymphoedema, bleeding, impaired nutrition and weight loss, sensitive and red skin.
- Long-term problems:
  - fistula, impaired healing, osteoradionecrosis (ORN), impaired swallowing, speech, and taste, xerostomia and radiation caries, loss of hair, radiation-induced tumours, neuropathies, cataracts, hypothyroidism, fibrosis.

Assessing chemotherapy patients:

- Short-term problems:
  - mucositis, nausea, impaired nutrition, weight loss, diarrhoea, bleeding, hair loss, neurotoxicity, immunosuppression, septicaemia, neutropenia, thrombocytopenia, multi-organ failure.
- Long-term problems:
  - nephropathy, cardiomyopathy, pulmonary fibrosis, ototoxicity, peripheral neuropathy.

Salivary gland diseases

- These patients are referred to the OMFS outpatient clinic by primary care doctors or dentists, or present with acute problems to the ED
- Salivary gland anatomy—see p. 26
- Acute salivary presentations—see p. 100.

Preoperative

History

If the patient presents with a lump, ask how long it has been present and whether it is getting larger. Is there pain and swelling at times of salivation (mealtime syndrome due to salivary obstruction)? Is there any facial weakness (CN VII involvement)?

Examination

- Lump/swelling: size, unilateral or bilateral, diffuse or localized, pain, hardness, tethering to deep structure or mobile.
- Specifically look for: whether saliva expressible from duct, neck nodes, oropharynx bulge (deep tumour). Test facial nerve function.

Investigations

Plain film, sialography, US scan, MRI (required to image deep to ramus), FNA (only serves to exclude malignancy; does not give diagnosis except if a cyst). Scintigraphy or sialadenoscopy may be useful.

Salivary gland diseases and their management

Salivary gland tumours

- The majority are in the parotid gland and are benign.
- Pleomorphic salivary adenomas (PSAs) are mainly found in the superficial lobe of the parotid and can be treated by superficial parotidectomy or extracapsular dissection.
- Monomorphic adenoma (Warthin's tumour)—benign, found in elderly.
- Lymphangiomas and haemangiomas are the most common salivary tumours found in children.
- Muco-epidermoid and acinic cell carcinomas are rare, and can behave aggressively.
- Adenolymphoma.
- Adenoid cystic carcinoma—more commonly found in the minor salivary glands and can be confused with mucocoeles when found on the upper lip.

Xerostomia

Causes—radiotherapy, drugs, anxiety, Sjögren's syndrome. Remove any causes, investigate for Sjögren's syndrome, and then treat symptomatically.

Sjögren's syndrome

An autoimmune condition causing xerostomia and keratoconjunctivitis sicca. It is sometimes associated with connective tissue disorders such as rheumatoid arthritis. These patients must be monitored for the development of MALT lymphoma (5% risk).

Diagnosis of Sjogren's syndrome

- Ocular symptoms (dry gritty eyes).
- Oral symptoms (dry mouth, frequent water intake, sticky tissues).
- Positive blood results—ESR, autoantibodies (RhF, SSA/anti-Ro, SSB/ant-La).
- Decreased salivary flow rate; sialectasis seen on sialography.
- Positive labial gland biopsy.
- Positive Schirmer's test, rose bengal score.

Causes of diffuse swelling of salivary glands

- Viral—mumps, EBV, CMV, HIV.
- Bacterial—acute or chronic bacterial sialadenitis.
- Sialosis—endocrine abnromalities, nutritional deficiency, alchoholism.
- Sialithiasis—diagnose with cheek (parotid) or lower 90° occlusal view (submandibular), although only 50% of stones are radio-opaque.
- Submandibular stones can be removed by intra-oral open or closed techniques or by removal of the submandibular gland.
- Parotid stones are removed by the intra-oral approach or superficial parotidectomy.

Mucocoele

- Common referrals.
- Submucosal cystic swellings caused by damage to the minor salivary gland or its ducts.
- Often a history of trauma to region.
- The lower lip is a common site—upper lip more likely to be a minor salivary tumour.
- Treated by excision of cyst and the associated gland under LA.
- Complications include reduced sensation to region as sensory nerve branches can be damaged.

Ranula

- A ranula is a mucocoele of the sublingual gland and its draining ducts. A plunging ranula passes through mylohyoid muscle and and can appear as a neck swelling.
- Excised by an intra-oral and/or extra-oral approach under GA.

Postoperative

Complications of parotid gland surgery to look out for

- Paraesthesia of ear lobe due to damage to greater auricular nerve.
- Haematoma.
- Salivary fistula or sialocoele.
- Temporal nerve weakness (10%).
- Permanent facial nerve weakness (1%).

Frey's syndrome (named after Lucy Frey, Polish neurologist 1852–1932)—gustatory sweating and redness over the parotid gland when eating. Caused by division of secretomotor fibres during surgery and inappropriate reinnervation of the sweat glands with parasympathetic fibres from the auriculo-temporal nerve. Can be treated with botulinum toxin injections.

Complications of submandibular gland surgery to look out for
- Submandibular scar.
- Haematoma.
- Weakness of the marginal mandibular nerve causing immobility of the angle of the mouth.
- Lingual and hypoglossal nerve damage—rare.
- If a stone has been removed, check that the gland is functioning and the duct is patent by milking saliva out of the gland.

Follow-up
- Any salivary malignancies should be followed up for at least 5 years.
- Benign disease should be followed up if treated by minimal techniques (e.g. extracapsular dissection for PSAs).

Orthognathic patients

- This is the subspecialty concerned with improving the position of the bones of the cranium and facial skeleton (*orthos*, straight; *gnathos*, jaw).
- The type of orthognathic cases that you see will depend upon the unit that you work in, but the general situation is that these are complex patients who require months of treatment (orthodontic), assessment (psychological), and detailed technical planning before surgery is undertaken.
- The management of these patients is undertaken at consultant level and within the context of an MDT. It is an ideal environment in which to observe the interface of OMFS with other specialties. You may be supernumerary in the clinic, so make the most of this learning opportunity.
- Patients will be seen at the joint clinic at various points in their journey:

Preoperative

Referral and initial assessment

- Identification of the main complaint (e.g. anterior open bite affecting diet). There is a spectrum of normality of the facial skeleton, and it goes without saying that people who fall outside the ideal dimensions do not need corrective surgery unless there is a significant problem, be it physical or psychological.
- Identification of syndromes (e.g. craniosynostoses in children may be part of the Crouzon's or Apert's syndromes, amongst others).
- Identification of patient's desires and expectations. Many strong features run in families (a famous example is mandibular prognathism in the Spanish royal family—'Hapsburg chin'), and it may be important to the patient to retain these characteristics. Their main concern might be having their teeth meet together.

Assessment

Examination of the facial proportions (soft tissue, hard tissue, and teeth) is undertaken systematically. The face is examined in the AP and vertical dimensions and any asymmetry is noted. Radiographs (lateral cephalographs) are essential to categorize the type of abnormalities found by measuring angles between various points on the facial skeleton. A classification will be given to both the malocclusion and the skeletal base which will dictate the type and amount of movement needed by orthodontics and surgery. The consent process should start here—patients need to be aware of the risks and benefits of surgery before they start a prolonged and expensive course of treatment.

Immediately prior to surgery

Surgery is undertaken after the initial phase of orthodontic treatment is finished. Make the following checks

- All the laboratory work (wafers for jaw movements) has been tried on the patient and has been signed off as satisfactory.
- Orthodontics have added hooks to the ortho wires for IMF.
- Preoperative tests are complete (bloods including group and save), and stop aspirin and oral contraceptive pill if possible.
- Ensure that any scans are completed and preoperative photographs have been taken.

Postoperative

- The orthodontic apparatus is left on for finishing touches after the surgery is complete.
- Check the occlusion (with elastics off) and assess the facial proportions (lateral cephalogram/DPT/photographs).
- Assess sensation—the IDN is vulnerable during mandibular movements.
- There is usually some relapse over time, so an over-correction is often made in anticipation of this.

Miscellaneous conditions in the clinic

Sinusitis

This is an important differential of facial pain. It is often worse on leaning forward (e.g. climbing stairs or wearing high heels). There may be post-nasal drip and purulent discharge from the nose.

Imaging is not usually helpful—fluid in the sinus and antral polyps are common and do not correlate well with symptoms. Rule out odontogenic and oncological causes; then refer to ENT.

Epidermoid and pilar cysts

These are very common (old term, sebaceous cyst) and are often found on the face or scalp where they can be multiple. Epidermoid cysts are from superficial layer of the skin and pilar cysts from the hair follicle, but in practice it is almost impossible to distinguish the two. The lesions are firm, well circumscribed, and tethered to the skin via a punctum (differential diagnosis lipoma, neurofibroma, turban tumour, etc.). When a cyst is infected it should be treated as an abscess, but formal excision should be arranged after the infection has cleared up.

Bat ears

The aetiology is a missing crease in the helix that is often hereditary, so be sensitive. Treatment is possible through various approaches but necrosis of the ears as been reported so consider whether it is really necessary. It is usually possible to obtain funding for surgery in children (although in financially conscious times this may change).

Pre-auricular pit

This is a congenital developmental condition. The pit can extend deeply into the parotid. The diagnosis may be made after an abscess in this region. Check the other side and perform MRI. Consider excision.

Skin tumours

- Some OMFS units specialize in skin tumours.
- Check the history for risk factors—sun exposure (sunburn at an early age is important), smoking (SCC of lip), and skin type. Check for industrial exposure (e.g. soldiers in the Far East can receive compensation).
- Look for other lesions—examine the parotid and cervical lymph nodes.

Thyroid tumours[1]

- High on the list of differential diagnoses of neck lumps.
- Check thyroid function and arrange FNA ± scintigraphy.

1 Koch W (ed.) (2009). *Early Diagnosis and Treatment of Cancer: Head and Neck Cancer*, Chapter 12. Philadelphia, PA: WB Saunders.

In theatre

OMFS operations

- OMFS is a relatively small specialty and often has to fight its corner in theatres.
- There is normally a theatre dedicated to OMFS, which may or may not be shared with other specialties.
- OMFS will have elective operating lists and usually semi-elective 'trauma lists', which should be consultant led to schedule trauma from the preceding week or so. In addition, there is the general emergency operating list where all surgical specialties list their emergency cases.
- It is common for some OMFS cases to have to wait to be done, as they are rarely surgical emergencies and more urgent (life- or limb-threatening) cases will go first. Ensure that your patient is kept informed and comfortable, hydrated, and pain free whilst waiting. Have a plan when to feed them if the operation is delayed to the next day.
- Although there is a wide repertoire of OMFS, a large part of the work in many units is dento-alveolar surgery. It is not surprising that most of the surgical errors in OMFS involve teeth (e.g. extracting the wrong tooth).

Tips for a junior trainee in theatre

Be confident

Theatre can be a daunting place for a junior trainee—lots of people with different roles, experience, and opinions. It can also be an inspiring and fun place to be. Don't stand in a corner and watch. Speak to people, ask questions, and make yourself familiar with every aspect. If you are interested and enthusiastic, you will be welcomed into the team very quickly, even if you feel that you don't know much. Consultants like enthusiasm and expression of interest!

Know your theatre etiquette

You need to be familiar with this before expecting to get hands on. Introduce yourself to everyone at the start of the list (now a World Health Organisation requirement), offer to help with the lifting of patient, and know how to scrub properly (if in doubt, get a scrub nurse to show you, as their technique is often better than that of surgeons). If not scrubbed, stay well clear of sterile drapes and don't get in the way. Ask questions at the right time, not when the operation is demanding the surgeon's full attention.

Be proactive

Ensure that the surgeon is happy with the preoperative marking of the patient, chart the tooth/teeth to be removed on the board in theatre, and ensure that imaging is available for the surgeon to view when scrubbed. Double check that the proposed operation corresponds to both the notes and the consent form. Ensure that all laboratory work required for the case is waiting in theatre prior to the case and is accessible.

Be a good assistant

- Keep your head out of the surgeon's light.
- Keep your hands out of the operative field.
- Do not grab instruments from the tray. Request them from the scrub nurse and wait for them to be passed to you.
- When suctioning, keep the operative field dry. Change to fine suction if necessary.
- Be gentle and careful with retraction—pressure on tissues can cause nerve injury (e.g. lingual nerve retraction during extraction of third molars, although this practice is going out of fashion in many units).
- Listen to and follow precisely any requests from the lead surgeon.
- Think ahead.

Be keen

As the junior, you may be supernumerary in theatre, but there are plenty of operating/hands-on opportunities. Team operating is often utilized in major cases, so there is often a place to stand, scrubbed, and assist. If you want to be a surgeon, being in theatre will be your future 'office', so get to know exactly how it all works.

Be efficient

In addition to your scheduled theatre days, bear in mind that it is normally possible to duck in and out of theatre whilst covering on call, and this is a good way to discuss the management of cases whilst getting hands on from time to time. This shows commitment and enthusiasm, and your effort will be appreciated. Try to complete TTOs or discharge summaries for patients in theatre so that there is no delay for the nurses to discharge the patient home if that is the postoperative plan.

Be prepared

If you are scrubbing for major surgery, prepare yourself physically for the long time you will spend scrubbed. It is reasonable to take toilet or food breaks during the very long operations. Do not be afraid to ask—there is often a team member who can switch positions with you.

- Know your anatomy and pathology
- Know your instruments
- Know how to write an operation note well

Overview of maxillofacial trauma surgery

Soft tissue trauma surgery

- The majority of small facial soft tissue injuries can be repaired under LA.
- Repair under GA if patient is a young child, or there are large multiple contaminated wounds or wounds that require significant exploration.
- Even under GA, a long-acting LA such as bupivacaine should still be infiltrated to minimize pain in the postoperative period. For complex wounds, it is better to infiltrate after the wound has been closed to prevent tissue distortion and incorrect closure.
- Contaminated wounds should be thoroughly washed and debrided within 24 hours. If there are deep abrasions with impregnated debris, they should be scrubbed to prevent permanent grit tattooing.
- With any soft tissue injury, it is worth remembering the reconstructive ladder.
  - Conservative treatment—leaving to heal by secondary intention.
  - Primary closure.
  - Graft:
    — split skin
    — full thickness
    — composite.
  - Local tissue flaps.
  - Tissue expansion.
  - Distant tissue transfer.
  - Free tissue transfer. 📖 See p. 164.
- Wounds should be closed in anatomical layers with an appropriate suture material. Non-resorbable monofilament sutures 5/0 or 6/0 are best for the face skin, unless their removal will be difficult (very young and very old patients), in which case use resorbable sutures (e.g. Vicryl Rapide).

Hard tissue trauma surgery

Generally performed under GA, although some simple dento-alveolar fractures can be managed under LA.

Fracture healing in facial bones is rapid and reliable and, unlike long-bone fractures, does not necessarily require rigid immobilization. There are two main principles of osteosynthesis for the healing of bony fractures.

Load-sharing osteosynthesis

The Michelet–Champy principles, introduced in the 1970s, described mono-cortical miniplate fixation, allowing a limited amount of micro-movement between the fracture ends while they heal. This has been shown to be very successful and is the principle by which most facial fractures are currently repaired in the UK. Titanium miniplates are lightweight and malleable, allowing bending and passive fit to the fractured facial bone ends. They come in various designs, widths, lengths, and thicknesses (e.g. 1mm, 1.2mm, 1.5mm, 1.7mm, and 2.0mm) which are adaptable to the various anatomical sites of facial fractures. 2.0mm plates are usually used in the mandible, while 1.5mm plates can be used for midfacial fractures. 1.0mm plates are good around the orbital rim. Titanium is well biotolerated and is designed to stay *in situ* indefinitely. However, for this method of osteosynthesis to be successful, the fracture ends have to be accurately repositioned and the healing conditions favourable, with much emphasis on restoring the natural dental occlusion of the patient. This may need to be enhanced with intermaxillary fixation in the healing phase.

Load-bearing osteosynthesis

Load sharing is only possible in optimum fracture healing conditions. If the healing may be compromised (e.g. by infection, comminution, previous radiotherapy, immunosuppression, diabetes, poor patient compliance), load bearing may be required. This may involve rigid fixation plates or bicortical fixation with locking screws, which completely immobilize the fracture ends. Reconstruction plates are used in edentulous mandible fractures as well as in head and neck cancer cases where the mandible has been resected.

Mandibular fractures

The majority of fractures will be treated by open reduction and internal fixation (ORIF) using plates and screws. Old-style treatment of jaw wiring may be used in difficult cases.

On the morning of surgery

- Liaise with theatre about what plating kit or wiring sets are needed and which teeth need extracting (angle fractures will need the transbuccal set).
- Liaise with anaesthetics as nasal intubation is needed.
- Bring any study models and arch bars, and put up X-rays.
- There is a risk of sharps injuries when using wires, so be careful.
- Document any pre-surgery lip numbness.

Michelet–Champy principles of fixation

- Facial fractures do not require rigid fixation for healing.
- Osteosynthesis can be achieved by application of load-sharing unicortical screws and titanium miniplates.
- Plates should be bent to passively fit the surface of the mandible.
- Anteriorly two parallel plates 5mm apart are needed to resist rotational forces.
- Posteriorly one plate is placed at the area of maximum tension, the external oblique ridge.

On the table

- Draping—head turban and prepare face if transbuccal is needed.
- Antibiotics given on induction.
- Although GA is used, most surgeons will also infiltrate with LA. A throat pack is placed (may be done by the anaesthetist) and direct vision gained by use of bite blocks and tongue retractors.

Operative

- All fracture sites are exposed by raising intra-oral muco-periosteal flaps.
- Occlusion is re-established. Patients are exquisitely sensitive to tiny alterations in their occlusion, whereas discrepancy of bone fragments can go unnoticed. If the occlusion is obvious, the teeth can be held together or fixed together with temporary IMF screws, arch bars, or Leonard buttons and wires. These can be left on to use with elastics postoperatively.
- This is a good opportunity to learn how to do the wiring. Take care that you do not cause a sharps injury! A useful technique is to make sure that the wire ends are always secure in the clips.
- Fractures are reduced carefully and may need to be held in place to allow fixation.

- Titanium miniplates are fixed with 2mm diameter screws through the outer cortex only, taking care to avoid the roots of teeth and the IDN. These can usually be applied through the flap, but at the angle where access is difficult the screwdriver has to pass through a small incision on the cheek.
- The assistant's role is to ensure that the surgeon has an adequate view of the fractures and that the plates are stable whilst being fixed.
- Flaps are replaced using absorbable sutures.
- Make sure that the throat pack is removed and inform the anaesthetist when this is done.
- In the operation note make a diagrammatic record of the fracture sites and specify the set used and screw placement.

Postoperative

- Ensure that postoperative radiographs are taken (OPG and PA jaws) prior to discharge (Fig. 6.1).
- Patients will need postoperative antibiotics, OH advice, and anti-bacterial mouthwash.
- They should have a soft diet for 6 weeks, which must be sloppy at first but can increase to firmer foods such as pasta and scrambled eggs after a couple of weeks.

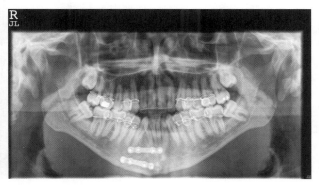

Fig. 6.1 Postoperative OPG of the patient shown in Fig. 4.1. The patient has had miniplate fixation of a right parasymphyseal fracture, conservative management of a left condylar fracture, and Leonard button IMF.

Complex fractures

Severely comminuted fractures or patients with poor-quality bone (e.g. edentulous mandibles, osteonecrosis, or osteomyelitis) pose a particular problem. Miniplates will not be sufficient in these situations, so much thicker reconstruction plates are used. These plates have to resist the muscular forces of the jaw and so are rigidly fixed with bicortical screws. Access is extra-orally under the mandible. Sometimes bone grafting (e.g. fibula) may be needed.

Condylar fractures

These can be treated by closed or open reduction. Open reduction involves an incision on the face and down through the parotid gland, so the facial nerve is at risk. Obtaining adequate vision can be difficult. Open reduction is indicated in bilateral, compound, and grossly displaced fractures. Closed reduction is achieved by intermaxillary fixation or elastic traction and can be used in minimally displaced fractures or where open reduction is not suitable.

In many instances, isolated condylar fractures can be managed conservatively. Even now there is controversy about the best way to manage these fractures.

Zygomatic fractures

On the morning of surgery

- Ensure that the patient is consented for ORIF zygoma with the use of miniplates and the possible approaches described.
- Risks include pain, swelling, infection, sutures, scar, retrobulbar haemorrhage (0.3% risk),and malunion or continued deformity.
- Patients should have at least two facial views available and may have had a CT scan.
- Marking the side of surgery with a marker pen is essential preoperatively.
- The anaesthetist may use an oral tube unless there are associated jaw fractures and the occlusion requires intraoperative assessment, in which case request a nasal tube on the contralateral side to the fracture.

On the table

- The tube should be secured and draped.
- The whole face must be prepped and left exposed, such that both zygomas can be seen (to compare), and the eyes protected with tape or shells if a transconjunctival or subciliary approach is to be used.
- Aqueous prep should be used for the face.
- Consider a perioperative dose of antibiotic and steroid.

Operative

There are generally three types of zygomatic fracture

- **Simple arch**—elevated Gillies or intra-oral approach; does not require fixation.
- **Depressed zygomatic body fracture**—needs intra-oral elevation or Gillies lift and fixation at the buttress. Advantage of the former is that there is no outside scar and the reduction can be directly visualizedwhile it is happening can be made.
- **Complex**—severely displaced, old, or panfacial fractures.

The zygoma tends to fracture at or near its three main articulation points—the zygomatico-maxillary suture, the zygomatico-frontal suture, and the zygomatico-temporal suture. If all three are involved this is termed a 'tripod' fracture. Orbital floor exploration may be required if the fracture is likely to propagate to this area.

- The aims of surgery are as follows:
  - to achieve facial symmetry
  - to achieve malar prominence
  - to relieve impediment of mandibular movement
  - to relieve orbital entrapment.
- A major cause of post-fixation instability is the masseteric attachment along the zygomatic arch (ZA) and body. For this reason, some surgeons electively plate all zygoma fractures (except arch) even if they appear stable initially following reduction.
- Fixation at the buttress (or elsewhere) is important to prevent late deformity.

- The lateral canthal tendon is attached to the zygoma (lateral orbital rim), so it must be fixed to prevent sinking of the palpebral fissure and an antimongoloid slant.
- Diplopia that fails to resolve suggests an internal orbital fracture and requires further investigation.

Gillies' lift

Incision 2–3cm anterior and superior to the pinna. Rowe's elevator is used to elevate the ZA out to its original position, which is usually stable. Appreciate the anatomy of the temporal fascia and relationship with the arch.

Open approaches

- Through existing laceration.
- ZF suture—lateral blepharoplasty, crow's foot, lateral eyebrow.
- Inferior orbital rim (transcutaneous)—subciliary, mid-tarsal, infra-orbital transconjunctival.
- Zygomatic buttress—buccal sulcus.
- Zygomatic arch—TMJ approach or coronal flap.
- Medial wall of orbit—Lynch incision.
- Complex upper third fractures—bicoronal flap.

Fixation

- Michelet–Champy priniciples apply
- Plates used are 2mm for the buttress, 1.5mm for the ZF suture and 1.3mm for the infra-orbital rim

Gems of knowledge

Anatomy of temporal fascia

This is relevant for performing a Gillies lift. The temporal fascia covers the temporalis muscle. Superiorly, it is a single layer, but it splits into two layers to insert on both the lateral and medial aspects of the zygomatic arch. Therefore the incision for a Gillies lift should go through the temporal fascia to allow the elevator to slide down and medial to the arch to elevate it out. It is important to realize that the fascia may have already split. Therefore incise through both outer and inner fascial divisions until you see temporalis muscle fibres.

Facial nerve frontal branch position

In the temporal region, the frontal branch of the facial nerve crosses the ZA and courses within the superficial layer of the deep temporal fascia. Watch out for the temporal vessels as well!

Postoperative

Because the zygomatic bone forms part of the rim and floor of the orbit, any displacement must involve the orbit. Consequently there is a 0.03% chance of blindness[1] due to orbital compartment syndrome at either the time of injury or postoperatively.

- Eye observations:
  - every 15min for 2 hours (pupil reflex, size and pain, tense globe and visual acuity)
  - every 30min for 2 hours
  - hourly overnight.
- Nurse at 45°, protect the side of surgery, and advise no nose blowing.
- Home next day.
- Follow up once in a couple of weeks after swelling has gone down.
- Course of antibiotics if preferred by surgeon.

1 Ord RA (1981) *British Journal of Oral Surgery* **19**: 202.

Orbital floor fractures

Orbital floor fractures

On the morning of surgery

- Ensure consent, including risks of swelling, pain, bleeding, infection, scar, ectropion, entropion, blindness (RBH), continued enophthalmos, or diplopia.
- Marking the side is again critical—mark on the forehead or cheek with an arrow to the relevant eye.
- Radiographs.
- CT scans with coronal re-formatting.
- Hess/binocular single vision (BSV) assessment should be available.
- If repair is delayed, a custom-made orbital implant may have been made on a stereolithographic model—have ready in theatre.

On the table

- A headlight is useful as in this surgery you are operating down a hole!
- Preoperative antibiotics/steroids.
- Eye shield with chloramphenicol ointment.
- Aqueous prep.
- Whole face exposed.
- Oral tube leaving mouth over chin (away from surgical site).

Operative

Approaches

- Transconjunctival
- Transcutaneous—divided by vertical level of eyelid skin incision:
  - subciliary
  - mid-tarsal/first crease
  - blepharoplasty
- Endonasal
- Transantral

Aims

- Reduction of scarring, ectropion, and herniated tissues.
- Free any entrapment and restore volume.
- Recreate and support floor of orbit using:
  - alloplastic
    - titanium mesh
    - Medpore
    - custom-made.
  - autogenous
    - bone—iliac, calvarium, rib, maxillary antral.

Surgical gems

White-eyed blow-out fracture

Paediatric orbital floor fractures due to springiness of bone. Bone fractures and springs apart, entrapping muscle and or fat before springing back up. This gives a tear-drop sign on the facial view (as opposed to a hammock sign). The patient may have an oculo-cardiac reflex with hypotension, nausea, and vomiting. This is known as a 'white-eyed blow-out fracture', as there is generally no subconjunctival haemorrhage. It must be repaired immediately to prevent muscle necrosis and long-term motility problems.

Anatomy of the orbital floor

Most fractures occur medial to the infra-orbital canal, which lies along the floor of the orbit. The part of the orbital floor least likely to be displaced is the orbital plate of palatine bone, which is located quite posteriorly. It is essential to find this by dissecting along the inferior orbital fissure (the only important structure is inferior ophthalmic vein which can be buzzed). The infra-orbital nerve is also close by and should be preserved whenever possible.

Postoperative

- Eye observations as with ORIF zygoma patients.
- Nurse at 45°.
- No nose blowing.
- Antibiotics/steroids.
- Home next day ± ophthalmic review.
- OMFS review (after orthoptics) 3–4 weeks.
- Removal of sutures by GP.

Other fractures

Midface fractures

On the morning of surgery

- Ensure radiographs, study models, and custom-made archbars are available in theatre.
- Consent for extra-oral/intra-oral approach.

On the table

Nasal tube may be difficult to negotiate with anaesthetists, but neecessary as dental occlusion is used to guide repositioning. Therefore the options are nasal tube, elective tracheostomy, or even submental intubation. Nasal tube is the best option.

Operative

The aim is to restore the bony skeleton to achieve normal occlusion and cosmesis. One of the hardest parts is trying to achieve the correct arch width when there is a palatal split, which is why custom-made archbars should be used for every midface case.

Frontal fractures

Two main types:

Anterior wall

- Generally a cosmetic indication if depressed
- Bicoronal flap
- Drains overnight
- Staples/sutures out at 10 days
- Follow up in 2 weeks

Posterior wall

- May need to cranialize the sinus if there is CSF leak. This is important to prevent subsequent meningitis, mucocoele, and Pott's puffy tumour.
- Discuss with neurosurgeons—may become a joint neurosurgical case.
- If required, ensure a bed on neurosurgical HDU available postoperatively.
- Drains overnight.
- Home with antibiotic cover.
- Staples/sutures out in 10 days.

Nasal fractures

- MUA is a fairly crude way of manipulating the bones.
- Primary open septorhinoplasty often required.
- Aims:
  - disimpaction of the nasal bones
  - correct deviation of septum and nasal bones
  - prevent nasal air blockage.
- External splint and internal packs at end of surgery.
- Nurse at 45°.
- Good analgesia.
- Remove packs next day and home if no bleeding.
- Follow up in clinic.
- Remove splint in 10 days.
- May require secondary or revision septorhinoplasty.

Dento-alveolar fractures

- Can be reduced under LA, but often better to do so under GA as it is distressing for the patient.
- Will require fixing with archbars or a rigid splint—ensure that the kit is available in theatre.
- Radiographs—OPG, upper anterior occlusal.
- Remove splinting at 4–6 weeks.
- Referral to dentist for follow up—may require endodontic treatment.

Dento-alveolar surgery

- Most common cause of litigation in OMFS.
- Spend time double checking radiographs, verifying treatment plans with the patient, counting teeth, marking sides, etc.

On the morning of surgery

- Consent must include the relevant dento-alveolar surgery risks of removing the wrong tooth, damage to adjacent teeth, IDN/lingual nerve injury causing temporary or permanent disturbance, oro-antral fistula, dry socket, infection, bleeding, swelling, trismus, fractured jaw.
- Have up-to-date radiographs available.
- For orthodontic extractions—copy of treatment plan must be in theatre to ensure that the right tooth/teeth are removed.
- Expose and bond—tell scrub nurse to have gold chain available or healing plates/Coepack for canine exposures.

Anaesthetic tubes

A nasal endotracheal tube (NETT) is best for the surgeon. A compromise can be made with an oral tube or a laryngeal mask airway (LMA).

On the table

- Supine
- Head ring to stabilize head

Operative

- Use of LA—best evidence shows that long-acting LA (e.g. bupivacaine) reduces postoperative pain.
- Antibiotics are generally overprescribed for dento-alveolar surgery, but their use may be considered.
- An intraoperative dose of IV steroid (e.g. dexamethasone 8mg in an adult) can be used to decrease postoperative swelling.

Removing a tooth

- Elevators or dental extraction forceps are adequate for most simple extractions.
- May need to remove bone with a drill or chisels.
- May need to section tooth with a drill or osteotome (the use of both chisels and osteotomes seems to be going out of fashion).

The concept of mucoperiosteal (MP) flaps

A mucoperiosteal flap improves access for bone removal around an impacted tooth. Design the incision so that the base is 2.5x length. Incisions must be placed over the bone and not the defect (think of the defect you might create!). You may need relieving incisions. Crevicular incisions are also useful.

The concept of removal of bone
- Coolant, suction, drilling, chisels
- Remove tooth
- Forceps, elevators, luxators, osteotomes/drills

Be aware of neighbouring structures, and ensure that the entire tooth is removed. If the root is retained, inform the patient and document in the notes. It is possible to electively leave roots behind in difficult third molar surgery (decoronation) by sectioning the crown. There is a small risk of subsequent infection requiring root removal.

Pathology
- Cysts can be enucleated after removing a bony window with the drill by peeling the lining from inside the bony cavity with a Mitchell trimmer or periosteal elevator.
- Marsupialization is an alternative option whereby the lining of the cyst is turned outwards and sutured to the surrounding mucosa.
- Always send any enucleated cyst or excised lesion for histopathology.

Closure
- Dissolvable sutures (except periodontal surgery).

Postoperative
- Painkillers.
- Paracetamol/NSAIDs; co-codamol 30/500 (📖 see p. 248).
- Don't wash mouth out for 24 hours.
- Hot salt-water mouth rinses—teaspoon of salt in a warm cup of water, held in the mouth for 1min but clean teeth with paste and brush.
- Follow-up not usually required unless complicated or a histopathology result needs to be chased.
- Ensure orthodontic follow-up for orthodontic cases.

Head and neck oncology and reconstructive surgery

On the morning of surgery

📖 See p. 180

On the table

- Depends on the operation
- Generally two teams operating
- Tracheostomy, dental extractions, tumour access (may need osteotomy), resection, ± frozen section, neck dissection, flap harvest, micro-vascular anastamosis, inset of flap, closure of neck and donor sites.

Operative

- Access and resection (may require lip split and resection of soft/hard tissues).
- Neck dissection—used for staging in clinically node negative neck (N0) or to remove metastatic lymph nodes. Blood vessel preparation prior to anastamosis.
- Raise flap (often at the same time as resection team), transfer and anastamose, microscopes, inset/reconstruct.
- Close donor site defect—may involve skin grafts (full or split thickness).
- Close neck ± tracheostomy.

Surgical gem

Spinal accessory nerve (SAN)

Knowing the SAN's course and anatomical relations is essential for avoiding iatrogenic injury during surgery to the posterior triangle of the neck. The SAN originates from the upper spinal cord as rootlets and roots forming the accessory nerve, which enters the skull through the foramen magnum, passing along the inner wall of skull before exiting through the jugular foramen along with the glossopharyngeal and vagus nerves. It heads inferiorly, piercing the SCM and sending motor branches, and then inferiorly to the trapezius muscle. It exits the SCM at the junction of upper and middle thirds, and passes back through the posterior triangle to enter the trapezius approximately 5cm above the clavicle. However, the SAN relationship can vary at this point.

Otherwise—learn your neck anatomy!

Postoperative

- ITU.
- Close observation.
- Drug chart—postoperative antibiotics, deep vein thrombosis (DVT) prophylaxis, proton pump inhibitor (PPI), steroids if appropriate, fluids, analgesia, flap management instructions. (📖 see p. 184)
- Stay until patient settled on ITU and all staff informed and happy with flap monitoring and any other issues.
- Monitor drains—their output over time and contents of bottles.
- Handover to the night on call—ensure postoperative bloods taken.

Salivary gland surgery

Surgery of the salivary glands is required for:
- benign neoplasms (e.g. pleomorphic adenoma)
- malignant disease
- stones
- trauma—complex facial lacerations.

On the morning of surgery

- Check consent. For parotid surgery, patients need to be warned about possible facial nerve weakness (temporary or permanent) to one or more branches and possible great auricular nerve numbness (earlobe and angle of mandible). For submandibular gland (SMG) removal, the marginal mandibular branch of the facial nerve (lower lip depressor), lingual nerve, and hypoglossal nerves are at risk of potential damage.
- Mark side.
- Liaise with anaesthetist:
  - nasal tube for parotid surgery
  - oral/nasal tube for SMG
  - **not** LMA.
- Liaise with theatre for equipment.
  - Stones will need an endoscope and a monitor stack.
  - Check if you require a facial nerve stimulator (disposable and expensive) or a nerve detection device (makes a noise when stimulated). NB: the anaesthetist should give short-acting paralysing agent only so that nerve function can be assessed.

On the table

- Position sandbag under shoulders.
- Prep whole face and neck. Drape with turban drape.
- Clean contaminated surgery, so antibiotics at induction plus 8mg of dexamethasone which has been shown to reduce nerve injury in the short term (presumed reduction of perineural oedema).

Operative/aims of surgery

Benign disease

Submandibular gland

Aim is to remove the gland completely through a natural skin crease, avoiding damage to the marginal mandibular nerve (which passes below the lower border of the mandible in just over 20% of patients). Remove as much of duct as possible to avoid stump syndrome and without damaging the hypoglossal nerve.

Parotid gland

Access via a pre-auricular incision which extends from the upper neck to the hairline. A skin flap is raised and the lesion/gland removed without damaging branches of the facial nerve. This can be a superficial/partial superficial or deep-lobe parotidectomy or extracapsular dissection. Avoid postoperative complications (e.g. sialocoele or Frey's syndrome (gustatory sweating due to aberrant reinnervation of the cut ends of the great auricular nerve)) although this is difficult to prevent. Extracapsular dissection is gaining popularity, Many perceived benefits including minimizing risk of Frey's syndrome.

Sublingual gland

Complete excision of a ranula or mucous retention cyst may require the entire gland to be removed. Lesions of this gland are less common than those of the parotid or SMG, but they are more likely to be malignant.

Malignant disease

- Parotid gland—surgery is usually conservative of the facial nerve if it is not already involved. NB: adenoid cystic carcinoma favours perineural spread and CN VII palsy may be the presenting symptom.
- SMG—malignancy may be diagnosed after excision, so careful surgery to avoid seeding neoplastic cells.
- Malignancy is proportionally more common in the sublingual and minor salivary glands.

Stones

Submandibular gland

Stones lodged in the distal or middle third of the duct can be recovered through the floor of mouth under LA. Those at the hilum or proximal portion need removal by an experienced operator under GA and an overnight stay as there is a risk of FOM bleeding. Have an endoscope at hand in theatre as it may be needed to locate the stone. Sometimes it is not possible to retrieve the stone, in which case the gland will have to be removed. Check that the patient has been consented for conversion to gland excision.

Lithotripsy is available in some centres.

Orthognathic surgery

- Check that consent has been done although complex surgery such as this should be consented by the senior surgeon.
- The main risk of this surgery is damage to one or more branches of the trigeminal nerve (inferior alveolar, lingual, infra-orbital nerves).
- There is a also a potential risk of airway compromise due to post-operative bleeding or oedema, although fortunately this is rare.
- These operations are usually bilateral so no marking is needed.
- Wafers will have been tried in clinic. Make sure that they arrive in theatre in good time for disinfection and use during surgery.
- Radiographs and study models also need to be in theatre and placed where they can be referred to during the operation.
- These procedures can be long, so make sure you have had breakfast and been to the loo!

On the morning of surgery

- Liaise with the anaesthetist—they will need a nasal tube and hypo-tensive anaesthesia. Antibiotics and steroids are given at induction, and usually continued for a couple of postoperative doses. Some units give tranexamic acid intraoperatively to reduce blood loss.
- Check your local policy on ordering blood units, but all patients will at least need a group and save and coagulation screen.
- Check that there is a HDU bed available. (some consultants request this although in reality most patients will usually be transferred back to the ward).
- Write clearly on the board what movements have been planned, e.g. 'mandible back 4mm with rotation 2mm to left, mandible forward 5mm with 2mm posterior impaction'.

On the table

- Position prone with head ring, prep and drape with head towel. Position the table head up.
- Double glove and wear goggles as there can be quite a lot of blood spatter.

Aims of surgery

Osteotomy of the jaws (controlled fracture along lines of weakness) to move them using the occlusion as a guide. The movements are planned around achieving a stable position of the teeth. This will have been determined by models taken near the end of orthodontic treatment. Hard acrylic wafers are then formed to fit the patient's teeth at each stage of the surgery to act as a guide for the surgeon. The fractures are then fixed with miniplates or screws.

Postoperative

- Patients will need to go to a high dependency ward with one-to-one nursing, as there is a risk of bleeding and airway obstruction.
- Loose elastics may be needed to achieve the final result. If the osteotomy has not been favourable, the patient might need tight elastic IMF.
- Make sure that all models etc. go back to the maxillofacial laboratory.
- Make sure that you arrange for postoperative radiographs (OPG and lateral view) before the patient is discharged.
- NSAIDs are very useful for both pain control and minimizing post-operative oedema.
- The orthodontist will continue treatment after discharge for 'artistic tweaking'.

Facial plastic surgery

There is a large overlap between plastic surgery and OMFS surgery with regard to soft tissue/cosmetic procedures. If this subspecialty is of interest to you, there are a number of aesthetic interface fellowship posts around the UK. Normally these are available for senior trainees nearing consultantship in OMF, plastic, ENT, and ophthalmic surgery. Further information can be obtained from BAOMS (http://www.baoms.org.uk).

With current and future financial constraints it is likely that the number of such procedures possible under the auspices of the NHS will be reduced to iatrogenic or post-traumatic causes. However, those who treat such patients will tell you that the psychological well-being imparted by even minor changes to appearance can mean that people crippled by self-consciousness can become successful (tax-paying) members of society.

It is important to set out realistic goals of surgery. Input from psychologists can be helpful, especially in diagnosing those with body dysmorphic disorder where surgery will not be helpful. Find out *exactly* what troubles the patient, e.g. nose too long, bumpy, tip deviated. They may be very happy to live with the aquiline nose as long as the tip is changed, so assume nothing.

Consent should be left to the most senior doctors. This is an area ripe for medico-legal cases, reflected by the high insurance premiums paid by those engaging in private practice.

Preoperative photographs should be taken in all cases (ideally by the hospital medical photography department).

On the morning of surgery

It is best practice to mark the skin creases when the patient is fully awake. This allows the incisions to be planned and agreed with the patient.

Operative

Local flaps of the face

Small lesions (e.g. BCC, SCC) can be replaced by local advancement or rotational flaps. Incisions are designed to remain within aesthetic units of the face whilst respecting Langer's lines, although in practice the defect and local tissue movement will determine the flap.

Rhinoplasty

This will be a functional/cosmetic operation. It is often indicated in cleft patients but is complicated by the fact that tissue may be deficient. Various courses are available to those who are interested in pursuing this field.

Blepharoplasty

In NHS practice this will often be undertaken after trauma where there may be problems with tissue deficiency. The main aim of surgery around the eyelid is to give a natural result without causing en/ectropion. There are specialist ophthalmic plastic surgeons who can help with surgery to these delicate tissues.

Scar revision

Always tell patients that it takes at least 12 months for a scar to mature fully (slightly shorter in children). There are various stages to healing where the scar will appear red, purple, and then white. Contractures can be avoided to some extent by massage with moisturizing cream or silicone preparations such as Dermatix® (may need prescription) or by triamcinolone injections. If the appearance is still unacceptable after a year, surgery may help. Make sure that there are clear objectives (e.g. thinner edges, level edges, flatter scar, elimination of dogleg, direction change). Promise nothing, especially if the scar is hypertrophic or keloid where special measures will be needed.

Filling defects

Injectable fillers or autologous fat (e.g. Coleman fat transfer) can be used. The long-term benefits are questionable.

Face-lift procedures

Modern techniques for improving facial contour are not based around tightening the skin, but involve tightening the superficial muscular aponeuritic system (SMAS) of the face. This is particularly useful in correcting facial nerve palsy, where a facial sling is created.

Brow-lift

This is usually an endoscopic procedure. Unilateral static brow-lift may be used following temporal branch of facial nerve damage.

Platysma placation

This done through small incisions or at the time of face-lift. Patients need to be warned about risk of marginal nerve weakness, although this is very rare. As with all aesthetic surgery, there is a risk of damage to one or more branches of the facial nerve.

Miscellaneous operations

Tracheostomy

This is not an emergency operation. If you need to secure an airway in a hurry, a surgical cricothyroidotomy is indicated (see p. 208). A tracheostomy is planned under controlled conditions.

Patients may be referred from ITU if they are slow to wean from respiratory support. Many anaesthetists can perform percutaneous tracheostomy, so those who are referred will be difficult (e.g. short fat neck, previous neck surgery, injury precluding neck extension). Make sure that you assess this adequately before theatre.

In theatre chose your tube before you scrub and make sure that the balloon inflates. Make sure that you have a good assistant. Incise the neck in a skin crease as low as possible. Deep to the fascia your incisions are in a vertical direction. Tie off the thyroid and its vessels to avoid major bleeding. Expose the trachea and stabilize it (e.g. silk sutures) so that it does not move once you incise it. Various incisions are possible—just make sure that you are below the first tracheal ring to prevent stenosis. Ask the anaesthetist to withdraw the tracheal tube whilst you insert the tracheostomy. Inflate the cuff and secure with silk sutures and a neck ring. Someone should auscultate to ensure that both lungs are inflated.

Cleft surgery

This is a subspecialty of maxillofacial and plastic surgery. There are only a small number of units performing cleft surgery around the country. This is because of guidance from the Clinical Standards Advisory Group that, owing to its complexity, this kind of care should be delivered by high-volume units only.[1]

In the UK many clefts will be detected antenatally. There are specialist cleft nurses who can advise parents about feeding and speech issues. When assessing the child, check whether the cleft is uni/bilateral and if it is lip and/or palate. Bear in mind unusual syndromes (look at general skeletal pattern and hands). The width of the cleft should be measured. All children should have a feeding and hearing assessment.

Repair is generally at 3 months for the lip and at 6 months for the palate. The downside is that some believe that growth is retarded by scar tissue when surgery is undertaken so early. The benefit is better swallowing and speech, and improved bonding with parents and siblings.

The chances of having a second child with a cleft are raised, so genetic counselling is indicated even if the pregnancy does not reach term.

There will be multiple issues through the early years such as missing teeth, nasal speech, poor hearing, and nasal regurgitation, and in all but the most minor cases multiple surgeries will need to be performed. Hence these patients are managed by MDTs including surgeons, SALT, orthodontists, audiometrists, dieticians, and psychologists. Many are in their early twenties before they are discharged by the cleft team.

---

1 http://www.dh.gov.uk/en/Publicationsandstatistics/Publications/PublicationsPolicyAndGuidance/
DH_4005945.

On the ward

OMFS on the ward

- Since OMFS is a small specialty with relatively few inpatients, it rarely has a dedicated ward and often shares with ENT or another small surgical specialty
- Sometimes the whole OMFS team attends the ward round, and may include 'special services' (e.g. Macmillan nurse, SALT, dietician, etc.)
- There are a large number of short-stay patients with no medical problems
- There are a small number of long-stay patients with many medical problems.

OMFS ward round essentials

- Pen torch, spatulas, gloves, elastics, skin marker-pen
- Stethoscope
- Hand-held Doppler for flap patients
- Review appointment cards if applicable
- Snellen charts for measuring visual acuity

Radiographs/investigations

It is important to ensure that radiographic imaging is available to be viewed on the ward round with the corresponding reports if completed. This is usually done via digital images on PACS (Picture Archiving and Communication System), often before the ward round. Be ahead of the game and have correct up-to-date images ready for the patient. Think about their interpretation and significance for management, as it is likely that you will be asked for your input. Furthermore, the latest blood, micro-biological, and pathological results should also be known and presented to the ward round.

OMFS ward work

A select few patients will take up the majority of your time (normally the oncology cases) as they require more regular investigations and post-operative monitoring (📖 see p. 184).

If you need to perform a procedure on the ward, try to make use of a side-room or ENT treatment room where you are likely to have more space, more light, and more equipment available than by the bedside. Ensure that you know the location of, and have had a play with, any equipment that you might need in an emergency.

Nurses

As ever, a good working relationship with the nurses is essential for a happy and harmonious working environment. Muck in and be helpful, and you will receive the same in abundance. Communicate well, share knowl-edge, and learn what the roles of the nurse involve.

Ward protocols

These are generally in place to follow in specific clinical situations. Some examples are given below'

Tracheostomy

It is useful to be knowledgeable about tracheostomies, so find and review the protocol (often in place for the nurses) for tracheostomy care. These guidelines relate to tracheostomy tube care, suctioning, humidification, care of the cuff, fenestrated tubes, speaking valves, decannulation, tracheostomy emergencies, and resuscitation (see p. 186).

Carotid blow-out

Ensure that you familiarize yourself with this, as the protocol is in place to decrease stress for both the patient and staff in what can be a seemingly horrific situation. The three approaches to carotid blow-out are preventative, active resuscitation, or palliative care.

- **Preventative**—prevent dehydration, infection, and wound breakdown; nutritional support; reduce physical and emotional stress.
- **Active resuscitation**—secure airway; prevent aspiration; control haemorrhage; prevent hypovolaemic shock; relieve anxiety; morphine/midazolam.
- **Palliative care**—relieve anxiety; compassion and support; assist the dying patient.

Alcohol withdrawal

This will be appropriate for a significant proportion of OMFS patients, particularly cancer and trauma patients who may be heavy drinkers. The protocol is designed to prevent delirium tremens and Wernicke's encephalopathy by administering a reducing regime of chlordiazepoxide and giving Vitamin B parenterally.

Likely ward referrals

Occasionally, OMFS receives a ward referral to review an inpatient under a different team.

- **Cardiothoracic/cardiology**—to screen for dental sources of infection, e.g. pre-CABG or stent, or if the patient has developed infective endocarditis.
- **Neurosurgery**—infective source of meningitis, brain abcesses.
- **Any specialty**—toothache referral. If you are not dentally qualified, know how to take a dental pain history, how to examine, and which special tests to organize before discussing the case with a dentally qualified member of the team.

Trauma patients

- Most of these patients will be waiting for either surgery or discharge. Occasionally you may have a multiply injured patient under another team that you keep under review.
- Continue to monitor airway, breathing, and circulation, as the status can change. FOM swelling caused by mandible fractures can develop late and you definitely do not want your patient to lose their airway on your ward. Do not just admit and forget about these patients—it has happened!
- Patients requiring neurological observations are not normally accepted by the OMFS team, so check with your senior before admitting to the ward.

Preoperative

- Make sure that your patient is put on an emergency list and consented. Get all imaging (remember two views for a fracture) and prosthesis such as splints and arch bars. Arch bars may need to be custom made if there are multiple missing teeth (will need impressions).
- Remember always to review the patient as other injuries come to light once distracting pain is removed or alcohol has worn off.
- The fixation of facial fractures comes quite low down the 'urgency ranking' of emergency operations. You need to warn these patients (who are not infrequently heavy drinkers and/or drug users) that it is likely that their operation will be delayed. Do what you can to keep them comfortable (e.g. withdrawal medications, methadone) and try to avoid self-discharge. You would be well advised to check liver function tests (LFTs), haemoglobin, and coagulation tests in these patients.
- Children usually have priority, and simple lacerations can be sent home from A&E to be brought back starved first thing in the morning for theatre. Liaise with theatre and the paediatric ward to ensure that space is made available.
- IV fluids are essential, especially if the fracture was the result of a drunken brawl. It cannot be pleasant to be NBM with a hangover! Dextrose saline is a good choice.
- Think about the situation in which the injury occurred. Is there a possibility of domestic violence? If so, this is a good opportunity to get help for the victim.
- Soft tissue injuries should ideally be sutured within 24 hours. You may need to press this point with the emergency theatre team.

Postoperative

- Most simple fractures can be discharged on the same or the following day.
- Postoperative radiographs should be checked prior to discharge (although the usefulness of this is questionable).
- Analgesia is usually in the form of NSAID + paracetamol ± codeine.
- Antibiotics are not normally required unless there is a compound fracture or delayed fixation.

- Facial lacerations severe enough to require GA will usually need review in clinic. They may need further surgery, such as scar revision, in the following months.

Mandible

- The occlusion should be the best indicator of adequate fixation. If there are obvious gaps between the teeth, let your senior know.
- Reassure the patient that numbness to the lower lip is normal and will usually resolve (document any pre-surgery numbness).
- Advise soft diet and avoidance of contact sports for 6 weeks.
- Oral hygiene is important. Brush teeth gently and use hot salt water and/or chlorhexidine mouthwash 2–3 times daily.
- Intra-oral sutures are resorbable. If an extra-oral approach has been adopted, make arrangements for suture removal (e.g. with GMP nurse).
- Review in clinic in 2 weeks and then after 6 weeks unless the patient requires elastics, in which case review may be needed sooner.
- They may require elastic IMF, and this may require adjusting before discharge.

Maxilla and zygoma

- Reassure the patient that it is normal to have a little blood from the nose. They should avoid blowing their nose for at least 2 weeks (wipe only).
- If a cranial flap has been raised, drains will be inserted in theatre and usually remain for 24 hours postoperatively.
- Always monitor for retrobulbar haemorrhage in zygoma fractures, both pre- and postoperatively (📖 see p. 242).
- Uncomplicated fractured zygomas are usually reviewed once at 2 weeks postoperatively.

Orbit

- Eye observations should be continued for 24 hours—the first 8 hours are critical. Look out for the three Ps of increasing Pain, Proptosis, or Pupillary defect, along with reduction in visual acuity which would indicate a retrobulbar haemorrhage.

Dento-alveolar

- Many patients with facial injuries will have damaged teeth and it is important that they are reviewed by a dentist once they are discharged. Give the patient a copy of any pertinent radiographs and a letter outlining their treatment to take to the GDP.

Dento-alveolar patients

- Most elective dento-alveolar operations are performed as day-case surgery. Patients who are not suitable for this (for medical or social reasons) may come under your care on the ward (e.g. warfarinized patients, haemophiliacs, children).
- Even if you are not dentally trained, it is inevitable that you will receive some ward referrals as the 'hospital dentist' and you will pick up the basics fairly quickly. Although you will not be able to replace lost or broken dentures, you should be able to assess a simple toothache!
- Abscesses in the head and neck region require a little more attention than elsewhere in the body, especially in children.

Trauma

Injuries to the primary dentition may require admission and GA as patients are generally too young to tolerate treatment under LA. Early loss of a primary tooth sometimes means that a balancing extraction of the same tooth on the other side has to be performed. This is to prevent asymmetric movement of the remaining teeth causing a shift of the centre-line and crowding which can hinder eruption of the underlying adult tooth. In the adult patient, teeth are frequently damaged during trauma and these are best followed up by the patient's own dentist. It is polite to phone or at least write to the GDP and to provide some radiographic evidence of the treatment.

Abscesses

Treat the cause as quickly as possible (i.e. emergency surgery as a priority case) as antibiotics alone will not arrest the infection (unless it is at the cellulitic stage before any pus has formed). These patients usually stay on the ward for a couple of days postoperatively and should have inflammatory markers checked daily. The swelling can worsen after theatre and some advocate the use of preoperative steroids if cellulitis is present. Check the drains (sometimes these are intra-oral) and chase any microbiology. Through-and-through drains will drain saliva as well as pus. The operating surgeon should make a decision on drain removal and shortening (warn the patient that it can be painful!). Sometimes patients need to return to theatre if they are not improving, particularly if there is a mouth full of rotten teeth, as it can be difficult to isolate the source. These patients, especially children, should receive some education in dental hygiene to reduce the chances of future infections.

Inpatient referrals

Some patients require dental review as part of their ongoing medical care. Examples are given in Box 7.1.

Box 7.1 Patients requiring dental review

- Endocarditis—assess if dental source of bacteria
- Extractions prior to major surgery (e.g. cardiac valves, transplants, IV bisphosphonates)
- Cerebrovascular accident (CVA) of infective cause—assess if from teeth
- Extractions prior to radiotherapy to the head/neck to prevent osteo-radionecrosis (sterile necrosis of bone due to ↓vascularity)
- Investigation of pyrexia of unknown origin

Assessment

- History—sharp poorly localized pain elicited by hot/cold/sweet food and lasting for a few seconds only can indicate pulpitis, which may be reversible if the cause (i.e. caries) is removed. Sensitivity on cold alone may be due to exposed dentine, resulting from over-zealous brushing. Pain which is spontaneous or lasts for a long time after the trigger is removed and is well localized usually means that the pulp is irreversibly damaged and should be treated by root canal treatment or extraction.
- Extra-orally look for lymphadenopathy or facial swelling.
- Intra-orally look for level of OH. Are there multiple restorations or obvious cavities? Are the teeth mobile?
- If the pain can be localized, it makes your diagnosis easier. Otherwise tap the teeth firmly (e.g. with a tongue depressor) and see if the patient jumps.
- Look for swellings and sinuses in the gingivae, buccal sulcus, and palate.
- OPGs are not very good for diagnosis of tooth pathology; a periapical is much better. If there are lots of crumbling teeth, OPG may be a lower radiation choice (see p. 42).

Head and neck oncology patients

- Approximately 50% of head and neck oncology patients develop a complication after surgery,[1] so they need considerable postoperative monitoring care on the ward.
- The patients are often unhealthy—malnourished and may be heavy smokers or drinkers.
- Expect the worst. As ever, prevention is the key.

Preoperative

- Patients are generally admitted the day before the procedure.
- Make it your job to ensure that the preoperative work-up/ investigations are complete.
- Check the clinic letters, initial assessment, staging, MDT discussion, proposed surgical plan, and preassessment investigations to gain a good overall knowledge of the case (📖 see p. 134).
- Consider PEG/RIG for postoperative feeding—often done before surgery.

In particular, ensure that the following have been completed:
- Cross-matched blood—check local transfusion protocols.
- Special free flap investigations.
- Radial flap—Allen's test (Doppler more sensitive). Record any pre-existing nerve dysfunction.
- DCIA flap—previous abdomen surgery (hernia repair/appendix)?
- Fibula flap—duplex run-off at the knee, CTA or MRA both legs:
  - Hip or knee problem on one side—use that side.
  - Preoperative nerve dysfunction—foot drop etc.
  - If reconstructing right mandible, left fibular is usually used because of its shape, although bone is usually osteotomized for best fit.
- Mark perforators—pen and hand-held Doppler.
- Ensure that the anaesthetist is aware that the patient is admitted.
- Imaging and histology available.
- Consent completed.
- Laboratory work prosthesis available.
- Fluids prescribed, if appropriate.
- Alcohol withdrawal (consider using chlordiazepoxide) and nicotine withdrawal prescribed.
- Laxatives prescribed (especially DCIA).
- Thromboembolic prophylaxis prescribed.
- Gastric ulcer prophylaxis prescribed (may be on steroids).
- Is the patient having a tracheostomy? Make sure that ITU bed is booked.
- SALT/dieticians should see patient preoperatively.
- Confirm postoperative feeding requirements.

1 McGurk MG, Fan KF, MacBean AD, Putcha V (2007). *Oral Oncology* **43**: 471–6.

Postoperative

Immediate—first 24 hours

- Likely to be on ITU.
- Think airway, breathing, circulation.
- Observations—pulse, blood pressure, respiratory rate, oxygen saturation, temperature, urine output.
- Tracheostomy care (📖 see p. 187).
- Monitor fluid balance.
- Flap monitoring (📖 see p. 184).
- Drains.
- Pain control.
- SALT/dieticians—PEG/RIG or NGT.
- Routine postoperative bloods—LFTs twice weekly.
- If on IV fluids—daily haematology/biochemistry in early postoperative period.
- If on enteral feeds, can often get vomiting/diarrhoea—liaise with dietician, change of feed may help.

Short term—first 7 days

- Regular observations and systems examination.
- Check for spikes in temperature, 'wind, wound, water, walk'—respiratory tract infection, wound infection, urinary tract infection, DVT.
- Tracheostomy—consider weaning (📖 see p. 187).
- Monitor flap healing—look for infection, dehiscence, fistula, delayed healing.
- Monitor neck dissection wound healing—look for infection, haematoma, seroma, salivary collection, chyle leak.
- Drains.
- Monitor donor site healing—look for infection, dehiscence, delayed healing.
- Try to remove indwelling urinary catheter, central line, IV cannula as soon as indicated.
- Routine postoperative bloods—LFTs twice weekly.
- Early mobilization.
- Chest physiotherapy.
- SALT/dietician review of swallowing and feeding requirements.

Longer term (>7 days)

- Head and neck patients can be on the ward for a long time.
- Common problems—alcohol and/or nicotine withdrawal, complications of malnutrition, chest infections.
- Keep bowels going—a regular laxative may be required.
- Remove stitches or clips depending on anatomical site.
- Consider arrangements for any adjuvant treatment.
- Social arrangements for discharge can prolong inpatient stay—find out about the patient's home circumstances and try to make early arrangements as required.

Drains

- Are they still working? What's in them and how much?
- Monitor the volume output over time.
- Look for blood, saliva (↑ amylase), or creamy coloured chyle (↑ triglycerides).
- Check that the drain is 'vacced' for as long as a vacuum can be maintained.
- Surgeons have their own preferences about shortening or removing drains. Make sure that you know what they are! If in doubt, ask before removing.
- If you take a drain out, 'de-vac' it before pulling to prevent discomfort.

Donor sites

- Radial—monitor nerve and perfusion, splint if composite (intra-operative plating).
- Fibula—splint, ankle at 90°, liaise with physiotherapist.
- Neck—shoulder physiotherapy to prevent shoulder drop.
- DCIA—catheter with Marcain.

Flap monitoring

- The purpose of flap monitoring is to identify a failing flap (usually a free flap, although pedicled flaps can also become compromised) at the earliest possible stage, to give the best chance of salvage.
- Flaps that return to theatre within 24 hours of surgery have a higher chance of salvage.[1]
- Pedicled flaps, such as the pectoralis major flap, may become compromised due to compression of the pedicle by the clavicle, soft tissue, or surrounding oedema or haematoma or by torsion of the pedicle at the time of surgery.
- Most causes of free flap failure occur at the anastamosis: venous engorgement (majority) or arterial occlusion.
- External and systemic causes are also possible—e.g. haematoma occluding venous drainage, low blood pressure, hypovolaemia, or arrhythmias.
- If there is no plan to return the patient to theatre if the flap fails, close flap observations are not required.
- Composite flaps take longer to raise, and there may also be greater blood loss during flap harvest.
- DCIA flaps classically fail slowly.
- Any concerns, inform senior EARLY.

How to monitor a flap

- Look for colour—free flap colour-monitoring charts can help.
- Palpate for temperature and texture.
- Assess capillary refill.
- Doppler assessment:
  - external hand held Doppler can monitor blood flow at the pedicle or main perforators within the flap.
  - some units have sterilizable metal probes for monitoring the flap intra-orally, or will have placed an implantable probe at the time of surgery.
- Prick the flap with a needle to look at the rate of blood flow and its colour (ask for senior help before doing this—generally only done to prove that the flap is failing).
- Microdialysis—sampling of tissue fluid for pH, lactate, pyruvate, and glucose using a probe inserted into the flap. Rarely used as it is expensive.

Monitoring regime

- Skin mark or stitch to mark anastamosis.
- Check flap hourly for 24 hours—colour and Doppler signal.
- Check flap every 4 hours for next 48 hours.
- Check with designated nurse that they are happy with the surgery that has been done, the normal colour of the flap, and where to place the probe.
- Do not be afraid to call a senior if you have doubts.

1 Brown JS, Devine JC, Magennis P, *et al.* (2003) *British Journal of Oral and Maxillofacial Surgery* **41**: 16–20.

Maintain good flap conditions

- Drains should have been placed to prevent collections in the neck.
- Maximize perfusion by keeping MAP 80–100mmHg.
- Ideal haematocrit is 30%.
- Ideal haemoglobin concentration is >10g/dl.
- May require pushing of IV fluids.
- Keep patient warm.
- Avoid tranexamic acid.
- No neck or flap compression with tight tracheostomy or neck ties.
- Try to prevent patient coughing.

Danger signs

First 48 hours

- Haematoma in neck—BAD
- Dark, blue, or mottled flap or very pale flap—BAD
- Dark flap with Doppler signal—BAD
- Immediate flow of dark blood on prick flap with needle—BAD
- Pale with Doppler—OK
- Very pale with no Doppler and/or no bleeding on pricking flap—BAD (rare)

Action required

- Patient resuscitation.
- Urgent exploration in theatre.
- Flap salvage—re-running of anastamosis.
- May require replacement local or pedicled flap.
- Venous engorgement can be treated with leeches.
- Close monitoring of haemoglobin and electrolytes.

After 48 hours

- Wound healing or breakdown around edges of flap—determines when a patient can start taking things by mouth, or when to take patient back to theatre to prevent communications between mouth and neck.
- The sequence that must be avoided is breakdown in the mouth around flap edges first, then sumping of saliva in neck, flap dies, and the neck bursts open.

Action required

- More sutures, pack, NBM.

The tracheostomy patient

- OMFS patients sometimes require tracheostomies, either electively for major head and neck procedures where the airway may be compromised or as an urgent operation if a surgical airway is required (although in an acute emergency, a cricothryoidotomy would usually be done first).
- A blocked or dislodged tracheostomy tube can kill a patient.
- Ensure that tracheostomy tube care is performed at regular intervals and that the tube is checked at every visit to the bedside to avoid sudden frightening blockages in the middle of the night.
- Tracheostomy emergencies (📖 see p. 234).
- Many hospitals have a dedicated tracheostomy nurse or conduct tracheostomy ward rounds, which are useful.

Types of tracheostomy tube
Can be a combination of the following.

Cuffed
- Inflatable cuff to prevent aspiration past tube.
- Used for all newly placed tracheostomies and for ventilated or unconscious patients.
- The cuff should have low pressure and high volume to prevent pressure necrosis to the trachea wall. Recommended cuff pressure is <25mmHg, and 5–7ml of air is usually enough to inflate it.
- When deflating the cuff, suction the oropharynx first to clear any secretions which may have pooled on top.

Uncuffed (plain)
- If no risk of aspiration, not ventilated.

Fenestrated
- There is a hole in the back of the tube which enables inhaled air to pass from the mouth into the trachea as well as through the tube placed in the neck. It can help a patient return to normal breathing or wean off a tracheostomy. It can also facilitate and improve speech.
- Must not be used if risk of aspiration.

Inner cannula
- Should be used with all tracheostomy tubes. The inner tube can be removed easily, facilitating the clearance of secretions.
- Prevents having to change the tube as often.
- Regular suctioning and humidification should still be performed.

Adjustable flange
- Used for patients with fat or swollen necks or a deep-set trachea.
- The flange can be adjusted to give the desired tube length to allow for variation in the distance from trachea to skin.

Accessories

Decannulation cap
- Used in weaning. The cap is placed on a fenestrated uncuffed tracheostomy tube to close it off, prompting the patient to breathe through their mouth. If the patient is managing to maintain O_2 saturations with this arrangement, decannulation is possible.

Speaking valve
- This valve allows air in through the tracheostomy tube, but not out. Therefore the patient can direct expired air up and out though the vocal chords and phonate. To prevent sputum blockage, do not leave on overnight.

Tracheostomy care
Aims are to maintain a patent airway, maintain skin integrity, prevent infection, and prevent tube displacement.
- Ensure the inner tube (if present) is being checked and cleaned regularly.
- Regular suction is required to prevent secretions from blocking the tracheostomy tube. Encourage the patient to take deep breaths before and after suctioning to maximize clearance from the lungs.
- Use a size 12 catheter to suction. About half the length of the catheter will reach the carina (often the patient coughs at this point) and then suction should be applied, withdrawing the catheter at the same time.
- Small volumes of sterile water can be syringed in to break up dried secretions or blockage, with immediate suction.
- All patients with tracheostomies should receive humidification of inspired gases via a heated humidifier, a heat moisture exchange filter, or nebulized normal saline.

Tracheostomy weaning
- A multidisciplinary approach should be adopted to assess the patient's gag and swallowing reflexes, dependence on suctioning, and physiotherapy to decide the best time to wean. There may be a ward or departmental protocol to follow for this.
- Absolute weaning requirements include a patent upper airway, a spontaneous cough, and the ability to clear secretions.
- Weaning methods normally involve increasing periods of cuff deflation, use of fenestrated tubes and speaking valves, downsizing the tube, or capping off the tracheostomy prior to final decannulation.
- Generally, increasing periods of cuff deflation until the patient has tolerated 'cuff-down' for 24 hours are followed by capping off for 24 hours. If this is not tolerated, the cuff should be re-inflated, and the trachea should be scoped to look for blockages.

Orthognathic patients

- Most orthognathic patients will be fit and healthy and in their late teens or early twenties so they usually recover fairly quickly.
- Generally this sort of surgery is well tolerated, and the preoperative planning is extensive so that patients will know what to expect.
- Swelling is inevitable, so nurse sitting up. Ice packs around the jaws and steroids can also help. They may be on HDU for the first night (although in many units patients return to the ward) because of the risk of bleeding/swelling compromising the airway, so take any calls about this seriously. Nurses are used to looking after these patients.
- They may be in elastic IMF and this may need adjusting depending on the postoperative occlusion. Elastics can be tight or loose. Class 2 elastics are placed more anteriorly on the upper arch. Class 3 elastics are placed more anteriorly on the lower arch.
- If placing elastics, arm yourself with eye protection, plenty of elastics, and preferably two instruments including a surgical clip and a pair of tweezers. Getting flicked in the eye with the patient's saliva, or indeed the elastics themselves, is not pleasant.
- The swelling can take some months to go, so warn the patient that the final result will not be apparent until then.
- As with any fracture around the jaws, the patient should maintain strict oral hygiene and a soft diet for 6 weeks.
- A couple of doses of IV antibiotics and steroids will generally be prescribed peri/post-surgery, although regimes differ with the surgeon.
- If there are drains, they should be removed after 24 hours if there is no excessive drainage.
- Patients will generally feel more sorry for themselves after the postoperative steroids are stopped. Generally, the best place for them to recover at this point is at home with good painkillers.
- The patient is followed up by the surgeon and the orthodontist, as the next stage involves 'detailing' post-surgical orthodontics, generally at 6 weeks postoperative.

Essential skills

Local anaesthesia

General points

- Maximum dosages are important and are covered in Chapter 11
  (📖 see p. 246).
- In this chapter we give practical tips on how to give effective mucosal
  and cutaneous anaesthesia with minimal discomfort.
- Use the finest needle you can and as few punctures as possible, so a
  long needle is better. Inject slowly, warm the solution, and give enough
  anaesthetic, especially for diffusion through bone.
- If you have to make more than two punctures in the skin, change the
  needle. The patient will notice the difference as it becomes blunt.
- If the skin is breached, inject into the edges of the wound from inside
  to avoid puncturing the epidermis. It is less painful that way.
- Wherever possible use regional blocks first followed by local
  infiltration afterwards if needed. This is useful for the haemostatic
  effect. (If so, wait 5–7mins for the vasoconstriction to occur!) For
  example, for a tongue biopsy, do a relatively painless lingual nerve
  block in the posterior FOM and then use local infiltration into the
  numb tongue for help with haemeostasis. Don't put the needle into the
  tip of the tongue first as this would be very uncomfortable!

The inferior alveolar nerve (IAN) block

This is also known as the inferior dental block (IDB).

- The aim is to block the IAN as it enters the mandibular foramen.
  This will render all the ipsilateral mandibular teeth, the lower lip, and
  part of the chin numb.
- It is easiest to do this with a special self-aspirating dental syringe, but
  this is not essential.
- Do not bend the needle. They rarely break but it does still happen.
- Open the mouth wide and with your non-dominant thumb feel for the
  external oblique ridge. At about 1.5cm above the plane of the lower
  teeth advance a long needle lateral to the pterygomandibular raphe for
  about 1cm.
- Deposit 0.5ml of solution there to block the lingual nerve.
- Turn whole syringe through ~60° so that the needle tip is pointing
  laterally and continue to advance slowly until you feel bone. Withdraw
  by 1–2mm. Before depositing the rest of the cartridge, gently press on
  the plunger to make sure that you are not in a vessel (blood will appear
  in the cartridge if you are). If so, reposition and try again.
- If you are using a non-aspirating syringe, you should aspirate first and
  check that you are not in a vessel.
- Now wait a few minutes for the solution to work.

Other LA blocks

You can block the mental, greater palatine, incisive, infra-orbital, supra-
orbital and supra-trochlear nerves by depositing some solution at the
respective foramina.

- The mental foramen lies between the apices of the lower premolar
  teeth and blocking here will render the ipsilateral premolar and incisor

teeth numb as well as the lower lip and chin. It is much kinder to block the nerve than to inject directly into the lip. You only need to insert the needle a few millimetres under the mucosa and the solution will reach the nerve.

- The infra-orbital foramen lies ~1cm below the inferior orbital rim in the mid-pupillary plane. You can approach it via the mouth or extra-orally. It will render much of the cheek, side of nose, upper lip, and ipsilateral anterior teeth numb. If you place your non-dominant index finger on the orbital rim and your non-dominant thumb inside the mouth in a pincer-like fashion, thereby elevating the upper lip, you will find that it is really quite easy to direct the needle to the right spot. Do not attempt to put the solution within the canal. There is almost no indication and you may inject intra-vascularly or cause a painful bleed.
- The supra-orbital foramen is on approximately the same vertical axis as the infra-orbital and mental foramina, and blocking here will render the temporal side of the forehead numb. Beware—the vessel which runs with the nerve is easily encountered and this block is rarely used for forehead lacerations. It is often less painful to inject into the wound edges. Similarly, the supra-trochlear block is not often used.
- The greater palatine and incisive nerves can be blocked, thus rendering the entire palate numb with three injections. This is often preferred as palatal local infiltration is painful. The incisive nerve lies in the midline just behind the upper incisors. The greater palatine nerve will be found about a finger's breadth medial to the very back of the upper alveolar bone. Ideally use some topical benzocaine cream first as these injections are painful.

Local infiltration in the mouth

- Depositing local anaesthetic solution under the mucosa and above the periosteum will render the overlying mucosa numb.
- In all areas of the jaws, with the exception of the posterior mandible, it will also render the pulp of the adjacent teeth numb by diffusing through the alveolar bone.
- This will not occur in the mandible distal to the premolars as the bone is too dense, hence the need for IDB or injecting into the periodontal ligament.
- They key to good infiltration is to inject slowly and remember that injecting into tightly adherent mucosa such as gingivae and palate will be very painful. Therefore you should try a regional block whenever possible, or inject from a numb area into a sensate area, thereby advancing the area of anaesthesia from an easy site into the difficult site.
- Teeth can be anaesthetized by injecting into the periodontal ligament. This is usually best done with a special syringe, but you can do it with a normal dental syringe. It is much easier if the tooth has periodontal disease.

Local infiltration for skin surgery
- Regional blocks are discussed above.
- When closing lacerations it can be less painful to inject via the open wound into the dermis, thereby bypassing the epidermis.
- Use as few injections as possible. A long thin needle which can be advanced as the anaesthetic is given is ideal.
- Dental anaesthetic and a syringe with a long needle is preferred by many surgeons.
- If you are anaesthetizing for elective surgery inject around the lesion in as few sites as possible in the dermal layer using a solution containing epinephrine, and then wait for it to work. You will see the skin blanch after ~7min.
- If you are removing an epidermoid cyst try not to inject into the cyst as it will cause it to rupture. Injecting around it may help by means of hydro-dissection.

Intra-oral suturing

General points

- Good patient positioning is essential for all surgical skills, but especially for working in the mouth. The patient can be sitting or lying down, but their head must be supported. You must have a good light source, suction, and an assistant, and you must be comfortable.
- You must be able to perform instrument tie. Practice it now.
- The main problem that beginners have is 'getting the knot down'. The key is to pull the needle end of the suture out of the mouth with one hand, whilst moving the needle-holders which are holding the free end of the suture down towards the suture line. However, it takes practice.
- Most intra-oral suturing uses resorbable sutures, but this is not always the case (e.g. when the wound needs support for prolonged periods of time: periodontal plastic surgery, over-implanted membranes, or closure of an OAF). In these instances a monofilament non-resorbable suture may be used, but these can be uncomfortable for the patient.
- Cutting or non cutting needles? Some favour one over the other.
- J-shaped needles can be very useful in places that are hard to reach such as the palate.
- Probably the best advice is to remember that the oral cavity is best approached through the front! This means that you may have to change the way you hold the needle-holders or position the needle in the tips in order to reach the wound from the front of the mouth.
- Suturing is a two-handed business. At times it may be easier to pick up the tissues with your non-dominant hand using forceps and place it onto the needle, so remember to use both your hands together.
- Don't always try to do it in one pass. You will often bend the needle or tear the tissues.
- Use the curve of the needle. Sometimes there will be a limited amount of tissue available and you may have only one or two tries before all tissue is damaged and unsuturable. Be aware of the cutting effect of the needle and think how the its angle of passage affects how the mucosa is pierced or incised.
- Don't think that you always need to close everything tightly. In most instances you just need to put it back where it came from. Open tooth sockets heal up naturally.
- If you are advancing some mucosa across a defect you may need to incise the periosteum only to allow it to move more freely. You will need long relieving cuts into the reflected mucosa and the sutures should lie over sound bone. Be gentle when cutting the periosteum or else you may have the separated flap in your hand!
- Try to avoid the mucosa pulling away around teeth, especially in the upper anterior region (the aesthetic zone).
- If possible, avoid having the needle coming out through the periodontal sulcus. It may worsen periodontal disease.
- The oral cavity heals well and is quite forgiving if you get the basics right!

Managing the bleeding socket

General points

- Sit the patient up; get good mouth opening; use head support suction, good light, and an assistant.
- Remove all of the clot and see exactly where the bleeding socket is.
- Is it the gum edges, within the socket, or is it from under a mucoperiosteal flap which was lifted to get the tooth out? The long buccal artery for lower third molars is notorious for this.
- If it is coming from under the flap, you may need to lift the flap up and have a look underneath.
- Consider the possibility that there is a medical issue. Ask about warfarin, clopidogrel, and aspirin, and manage accordingly. Has the patient taken metronoidazole postoperatively with their warfarin? Remember, this raises the INR.
- Give plenty of LA—a regional block first and then, using a solution containing epinephrine (adrenaline), give a lot around the site including the socket edges and wait for at least 7min for the homeostatic effect to work. During this time the patient can bite on a pack.
- If there are sutures and/or a packed socket already, remove them and start again.
- Clean the socket and pack it with resorbable cellulose (Surgicel®).
- Suture the socket tightly with a horizontal mattress suture of 3.0 braided resorbable suture or black silk.
- Apply a pressure pack over the socket and ask the patient to bite down on it for 30min.
- During this time you can recheck their observations and do any medical jobs you may need to do, like checking their INR.
- In almost all cases this is adequate.
- Consider tranexamic acid.
- Don't assume that a tooth socket cannot be a major source of blood loss. It can, and in some patients it could be fatal. Treat them in the same as you would any other bleeding patient.

Suturing the bleeding socket

- The purpose is to compress the gum edges against the bone edges and to hold the resorbable cellulose pack in place.
- A horizontal mattress suture in 3.0 braided resorbable suture or black silk is best.
- It must be tight, so take good-size bites.
- This may require you to mobilize some of the attached gingival tissue around the socket—literally lift it up so that you can get under it for a couple of millimetres with a periosteal elevator, especially on the lingual or palatal side. However, it is time well spent to get this stage right.
- A couple of interrupted sutures will also do, but if it is not tight take it out and do it again. If you are struggling to keep the tension on, try hand tying.

Managing the dry socket

General points

- This is also known as localized osteitis.
- A dry socket is one that is not healing and is extremely painful.
- The normal blood clot within the socket (which is the first step of the normal healing process) has been lost, possibly because of anaerobic bacterial action and food debris collected in the empty socket. The bone of the socket is exposed and painful to touch, there may be some degree of inflammation of surrounding soft tissues, the smell is unpleasant, and the patient may have trismus in the bone.
- It usually presents about 3–4 days after extraction.
- Giving perioperative antibiotics probably does not make any difference, and post-operative definitely doesn't, so don't blame the dentist.
- It is most common in the lower third molar area, in women on OCP and smokers, and possibly after periodontal ligament injection.
- Not everyone who presents with pain and swelling after dental extractions has a dry socket, so always examine them fully and check that they have not got an abscess somewhere. In particular, look out for pus on the lingual side or around the pharynx as this can be life-threatening.
- Consider other possibilities. Is there a fragment of tooth or bone that has been left behind in the socket? Is there a fracture through the socket which may have occurred perioperatively or post operatively? If you think so get a radiograph.

Treatment

- It may be helpful to give an IDB but this is not always necessary.
- Irrigate the socket with copious warm saline to remove all the food debris.
- If you have a good IDB, you can scrape the lining of the socket to encourage bleeding and remove the non-vital bone.
- In most cases it is kinder and just as effective to pack the socket with Alvogyl (see p. 252) or a similar substance.
- Antibiotics are not indicated unless there is evidence of systemic infection or significant local inflammation of the soft tissues, or the patent is immunocompromised.
- NSAIDs are sufficient for the pain which usually settles quite quickly after Alvogel is placed.
- One visit is usually enough, but occasionally further packing may be needed.

Suturing facial lacerations

General points

- Make sure that you are not missing an underlying facial (or skull) fracture. The classic is a chin laceration with associated condylar fractures.
- Look for facial nerve injury before you put in LA.
- Most minor facial lacerations can be closed quickly in A&E under LA and no follow-up is required.
- The more serious lacerations require special attention. If you are seeing them in the middle of the night, it may be better to dress the wound and bring them back to a clinic the next day when you have better facilities in your outpatient department and more help.

Wound preparation

- Clean the wound with copious saline.
- Give LA—a combination of regional blocks and local infiltration into wound edges is usually ideal.
- Remove any debris and irrigate again.
- Excise non-vital tissue and crushed wound edges so that the wounds are clean and incised at 90° to the skin surface.

Suturing

- Align anatomical borders, such as vermilion, brow, and eyelid, first.
- If there is skin loss, surgery is becoming tricky. Call your senior.
- For deep layers use resorbable sutures (e.g. 4/0 Vicryl or Maxon) to close the dead space and take some tension off the skin edges.
- If the laceration is a straight line, a continuous dermal suture may be ideal. This could be a resorbable or non-resorbable monofilament.
- Use 5.0 or 6.0 non-resorbable monofilament suture for most skin sutures. In small children a 6/0 or 7/0 resorbable suture may be better to avoid the need for sedation or GA to remove sutures.
- Sutures on the face can be removed at 5 days.
- If the wound is not gaping or the deep sutures hold the skin edges together well, you may be able to use a dermal adhesive as long as you are familiar with the product. Don't get it in the eye. Don't use it with a non-compliant patient and don't get it in the wound! It acts as a bridge across the wound surface by sticking to the skin on each side of the wound. It also acts as a barrier to fluid, so once it has set the wound is watertight. Advise the patient to apply white soft paraffin to the glue after about 7 days and definitely not to pick at the glue.
- A laceration which is clean and not gaping may only need Steri-Strips™.

Lip lacerations

- Check if the laceration is full thickness. In punching injuries and falls the lip may be pushed against the tooth, so check for an associated dental or bony injury.
- Mental nerve blocks are kind. Local infiltration afterwards may help haemostasis.
- Align the vermilion border first.
- Suture the muscle and then the mucosa, both with resorbable sutures.
- Close the skin last.

Ear lacerations

- Look for a perichondral haematoma—if untreated, this leads to cauliflower ear, so if you find it drain it! A small stab incision under LA will allow drainage.
- Exclude base of skull fractures and examine the external auditory meatus.
- Wash well and close the skin over the cartilage with non-resorbable sutures.
- You may need a pressure dressing for 24 hours.

Eyebrow lacerations

- Align the tissue carefully.
- Excise non-vital tissue parallel to the hair shafts.
- Never shave or cut the hairs.

Eyelid lacerations

- Exclude globe injuries. Discuss with the ophthalmologist.
- Look for damage or rupture to levator palpebrae superioris.
- Does laceration involve the lacrimal apparatus? If so, you will definitely need help. Call your senior and the ophthalmologist.
- Align the tarsus carefully.
- Eyelid skin heals well, so you can be minimalist with your suturing.

Nose lacerations

- Check for a septal haematoma and drain it if you find it.
- If laceration is full thickness, close the mucosa first.
- Align skin, especially around the alar margin, and close with non-absorbable sutures.
- Lost tissue is a 'call senior' moment. It is often treated conservatively initially, especially if the wound is dirty.

Packing the nose and midface for bleeding

General points

- Some of this is covered in Chapter 10, but it is important and so there may be some duplication.
- Patients die because of inadequate resuscitation and delay in treatment.
- In this chapter we deal only with the techniques. Knowledge of the general management of bleeding patients is expected and specifics are covered in Chapter 10.

Packing the nasal cavity

- Sit the patient forward and pinch nostrils.
- Whilst they are sitting there, explain that you are going to place a couple of tampons in their nose which will stop the bleeding.
- Explain that it will be uncomfortable briefly but you will do it quickly.
- Get two nasal tampons and lubricate the end that does not have a string attached with plenty of water-based lubricant.
- If the patient is sitting they must have head support, it may be easier to do this with them lying down briefly.
- Lift up the nose tip and in one brisk firm movement push the tampon backwards along the nasal floor parallel to the hard palate.
- The tampon is a bit like a lolly stick! The flat surface should be parallel to the nasal septum.
- It may be necessary to insert one on each side.
- They should not normally be left *in situ* for more than about 24 hours.
- The strings can be tied together and a bolster placed under the nose.

Packing the midface

- If safe to do so, sit the patient up and allow them to lean forward.
- Get a good light source and suction out the mouth and anterior nose.
- Try to find the source of bleeding.
- Pass a Foley catheter along the nasal floor so that the balloon is just beyond the posterior nasal aperture and inflate the balloon. Repeat on other side.
- Pull the inflated balloons against the posterior nasal aperture and then pack the anterior nasal cavity with nasal tampons on both sides.
- Use a disposable drain clamp to secure the Foley catheter and maintain pressure.

Re-implanting and splinting teeth

General points

- The socket must be adequately anaesthetized, so give injections as if you were taking the tooth out.
- Make sure that it really is a permanent tooth. There is no reason to re-implant a deciduous tooth!
- Re-implantation is most likely to be successful in young people who have presented within an hour or two with a tooth which has been kept in saliva, saline, or milk.
- Do not attempt re-implanting a tooth which has been out for hours and is dry and dirty. It is not a pleasant procedure and in such cases it will not work anyway.
- If you are not dentally qualified, try and get someone who is to help you.
- Time is the major factor determining success, so it cannot wait until the morning.
- Give the patient a short course of broad-spectrum antibiotics and regular simple analgesia.
- After re-implantation or reduction of a displaced tooth, it is usually necessary to splint it.
- The patient will need a follow-up the next day with a dentist.

Re-implanting or repositioning a tooth

- Hold the tooth by the crown and gently rinse it in sterile saline. Do not touch the root surface at all.
- Ensure that you have the right tooth for the right hole. This can be difficult if both central incisors have been lost, but if you look carefully at someone else (e.g. the patient's partner) as a guide, you will see the subtle differences with the incisive slant—the distal part (towards the back of the mouth) looking from the front has more of a curve at the incisal edge than the medial edge (towards the front).
- Make sure that the socket is clean and empty, give LA, and irrigate the socket.
- Firmly push the tooth back into the socket. Then place a gauze pack between the upper and lower teeth and ask the patient to bite on it in such a way as to hold the tooth in the socket. You will now need to splint the tooth.
- Repositioning the tooth is much same. You need lots of LA and you physically move the tooth back to correct position and splint it.

Splinting teeth

There are many ways of splinting a tooth Get someone to show you one and practice it. Most use a wire and some composite resin, or a glass ionomer that sticks to dry tooth enamel. When you have mixed it, put it on the labial side of the tooth with two teeth either side, and place a pre-bent orthodontic wire into the material. Put some more over the wire and wait for it to set! It's really quite easy!

Temporomandibular joint relocation

General points
- Patients will present with an inability to close the mouth, pain, and drooling.
- It may follow yawning, trauma, dentistry, vomiting, or anaesthesia.
- If there is anything in the history to suggest that there could be a fracture, you should get radiographs, but these are not usually needed to diagnose a dislocated mandible.
- If the patient can close their teeth together, the TMJ cannot be dislocated, but they may have a displaced temporomandibular disc which is another matter entirely.
- If possible, sit them in a chair so that their head is at your elbow height.
- Stand in front of them and place the thumbs of both hands inside the mouth on the bone lateral to the mandibular molar teeth as far back as possible, with your fingers supporting the lower border.
- You are going to close the mouth whilst pushing down on your thumbs.
- Keeping your arms straight, lean forward and push down and backwards (backwards for the patient that is) using your body weight onto your thumbs in a slow controlled fashion whilst rotating your wrists and pushing under the jaw in an upwards direction with your fingers.
- You may find that one side goes in first, and if you continue the action the other side will 'clunk' in place.
- An alternative technique is to place a 5ml syringe across the posterior-most molars and advise the patient to bite together whilst you push upwards from under the chin.
- If this fails, which is more common if the jaw has been dislocated for more than a couple of hours, it may be necessary to relocate under sedation or GA.
- Be very cautious about giving sedation in the ED for this problem. Talk to your senior first.
- Recurrent dislocation can be a nuisance, and sometimes it is worth showing the patient's partner or carer how to relocate the mandible.
- A follow-up appointment is usually worthwhile.

Bridle wiring and intermaxillary fixation

General points

- Sharps injuries from wires are more common than they should be, so be careful. Never leave a wire sticking out of the mouth. It must have an instrument on the end.
- Bridle wiring can help support a fracture and reduce pain.
- IMF is useful for reducing a fracture, immobilizing a fracture, or just guiding the mandible in function during the healing phase. It can vary from a rigid IMF to minimal guidance.

Placing a bridle wire

- This is usually best done under LA.
- Use 0.45mm pre-stretched stainless steel wire.
- Using an appropriate wire-holding instrument (heavy clip) push the wire between the teeth so that it goes around at least one tooth on each side of the fracture and both ends come out on the labial side of the mouth.
- Using both clips wrap the wires once around each other in a clockwise direction.
- Now place one clip on both wires where they are wrapped around each other and pull the wire towards you. Then, without pulling, gradually tighten the wire by turning the clip clockwise. You should see the wire wrap around itself and the fracture will be reduced and immobilized.
- Beware of loose teeth which can be extruded using this technique.

Intermaxillary fixation

- The eyelet wires, IMF screws, or Leonard buttons are usually put on under GA, and that is the best time for you to learn the technique.
- Orthognathic and some trauma patients may have some IMF using orthodontic appliances
- You may be asked to put a patient into IMF who has IMF screws, Leonard buttons, or orthodontic braces.
- This is usually done with special orthodontic elastic bands which come in packets of different colours depending on their strength. Red seems to be a favorite in OMFS.
- When you are asked, you need to know how tight and what direction.
- Force will be light, moderate, or rigid.
- The direction is as follows:
  - class III elastics are positioned to have vector of force pulling the chin backwards
  - class II is the opposite
  - class I is neutral.

Incision and drainage of intra- and extra-oral abscesses

General points

- Every patient with an abscess must have a blood sugar measurement. It is always worth looking for undiagnosed diabetes!
- If the patient is to be admitted, get WCC and CRP.
- You must answer the following questions.
  - What is the source of the abscess (tooth, skin cyst etc)?
  - What is the extent of the abscess?
  - Does the patient have any underlying medical problems—diabetes, immunocompromise?
  - Can the abscess be dealt with adequately under LA?
  - Is the patient systemically unwell or is there an airway risk?

Simple intra oral abscesses

- Inject a small amount of LA intra-mucosally at the point of maximum convexity of the abscess.
- This may be less painful if the needle approaches from the side.
- When the overlying mucosa is blanched, quickly incise it with a No 11 blade and send a pus sample for microbiology culture and sensitivity.
- On the palate it may be necessary to excise a window of mucosa to allow further drainage or use a small Penrose drain.
- Treat the source of the abscess. Is there a tooth which needs removing or a root filling?
- An alternative is the raise a mucoperiosteal flap. This usually warrants a Penrose drain.

A few other points

- Maxillary sinus cancer may erode through the palate and present as a palatal abscess.
- You will rarely be criticized for putting a drain in, but eventually there will be a time when you didn't, and then you will wish you had!
- If you don't treat the source of the infection, it will usually come back.
- Upper lateral incisors often discharge to the palatal side.
- The canine fossa is an intra-oral site on a latitude with the nostril. Pus from the canines and incisors accumulates their and you may need to drain this site using an intra-oral approach. It is a lot farther up than most people realize and hence inadequate drainage is common—but now you know that you will avoid making that mistake!

Simple skin abscesses

- These are usually secondary to folliculitis or inflamed epidermoid cysts.
- They can usually be incised and drained with a small amount of LA into the overlying skin or an injection into the skin around the abscess as described above.
- Sometimes a spray with ethyl chloride (wait until skin blanches) and a quick stab is sufficient.
- Always use a drain—Penrose or Wick is the usual choice.
- Always get a pus sample and describe what you find in the notes. Is it a 'cheesy' substance?
- Put a dressing on and bring the patient back to clinic in about 4 days.
- If there is surrounding cellulitis always consider giving antibiotics.

Complex head and neck abscesses

- Some head and neck abscesses require drainage through the skin under GA.
- These are usually collections in the submandibular, submental, sub-lingual, and parapharyngeal spaces.
- Most common causes are dental and salivary gland abscesses.
- The patient needs admission, FBC, CRP, random glucose, IV antibiotics, and fluid resuscitation. Some advocate dexamethasone (always get senior advice before starting this yourself).
- Try to determine the source of the infection. It will often be dealt with at the time of drainage, especially if dental in origin, so you may need an OPG.
- Keep patients NBM and get an airway assessment quickly if you think that there is any risk to airway competence.
- If they have trismus the anaesthetist may have trouble intubating and will usually want to get the case done in daylight hours (often using the fibreoptic intubation technique), so inform them straight away. Even if there is no airway compromise, these patients can still present an intubation problem.
- For management of airway compromise see p. 232.

Biopsy of intra- and extra-oral lesions

General points

- Most biopsies will be either incisional or excisional.
- The most common fault with biopsies is not giving the pathologist enough clinical information—fill the form in fully.
- If you are sending something which is visible on a radiograph, it is sometimes worth sending a copy.
- If you are doing an incisional biopsy, ensure that you get a piece of reasonable size and don't crush or tear it.
- If you suspect cancer mark it as urgent.
- For oral blistering conditions you may need a special transport medium (Michel's) for immunofluorescent tests. Ask the laboratory first.
- Do not do an incisional biopsy of a melanoma unless you have been told to do so. It is usually inappropriate except in some delicate anatomical areas or in cases of suspected lentigo maligna.
- If there is any possibility that you are about to cut into a vascular lesion, put a needle into it first to see. High-flow vascular malformations bleed copiously and can be difficult to stop.
- Use diagrams and consider photography.
- Histopathology will not always give you the diagnosis. Sometimes it also needs a good old history and clinical examination.

Biopsy of mucosal lesions

- Inject a small amount of LA under or around the lesion, never into it or else it will damage the architecture and may make diagnosis difficult.
- Excise an ellipse with the long axis running postero-anteriorly.
- Close with a couple of interrupted resorbable sutures. You can invert them to avoid any loose ends.
- For incisional biopsies include a representative sample and make sure that you are not just excising a necrotic area which will not be diag-nostic. Biopsying from the edges of the lesion is usually ideal.

Biopsy of skin lesions

- Think about where the scar will run. Try to hide it in a skin crease.
- Prepare the skin with a cleansing agent.
- Do not operate on broken or inflamed skin, unless that is the reason for the biopsy. It is more likely to become infected and heal badly.
- If you are taking a sample of a diffuse area or the edge of a suspicious lesion, consider punch biopsy. It is quicker.
- If you will not be able to get primary closure, it is best to talk to your senior before you start!
- Refer to British Association of Dermatology guidelines for margins of malignant lesions (3–4mm for nodular BCC, 1cm for SCC, etc.). Unless you are very familiar with this practice, it is advisable to talk to your senior.
- You should have a bipolar diathermy to hand.

Minor salivary gland biopsy

- This is usually for the diagnosis of Sjögren's syndrome.
- Ask your assistant to squeeze the lower lip at the corners bilaterally and evert the lower lip somewhat as well. This reduces bleeding and makes access much easier.
- Incise the lower lip mucosa vertically. Do not extend onto the skin.
- The minor salivary glands will burst out of the wound like tiny grapes.
- Remove five minor salivary glands and send them in formalin—don't go foraging around. You can damage the delicate sensory nerves, resulting in a numb patch over the biopsy site.
- Close with a couple of interrupted resorbable sutures.
- Make sure that you tell the histopathologist that you are looking for a diagnosis of Sjögren's syndrome.

Temporal artery biopsy

- This is usually for cranial arteritis.
- Palpate the anterior branch of the superficial temporal artery and mark its course on the skin. It often goes into spasm when the LA is infiltrated and can then be harder to find.
- Inject LA into the dermis in a 5cm radius around the artery and wait for the skin to blanch.
- There should be no need to shave the skin, but you should prepare it with a cleansing solution.
- Make an incision within the hairline, parallel to the hair shafts over the artery just through skin. The artery is deep to skin and there is no need to worry about cutting into it if you are careful.
- Using a couple of 'cat's paw' retractors. Ask your assistant to retract the skin on both sides.
- Bluntly dissect through the dermis and subdermis carefully, opening the tissues with an artery clip.
- When you find the artery choose a 2cm long piece and tie and cut it at both ends.
- Send it in formalin, making it clear you are looking for cranial arteritis.
- Close with a few interrupted sutures of your choice.

Biopsy of intra-bony lesions

- Beware of high-flow vascular malformations. Massive bleeding is quite possible.
- Wherever possible raise a muco-periosteal flap from the gingival margin with one or two relieving incisions.
- You may find that the lesion has perforated the bony cortex, but if it has not remove some overlying bone with a round burr.
- If it is likely to be a cyst, aspirate some fluid using a needle and syringe and send that separately. Get a good sample of the cyst lining, taking care not to damage the IAN or tooth apices.
- Close the flap over the defect.

Nasendoscopy

If you have done an ENT job you will not need to read this section.

General points and technique

- Sit the patient in a chair with head support.
- Tell them you are going to put a small tube up their nose so you can see down their throat, and it is uncomfortable and they will feel as if they have a head cold for a while afterwards.
- Check that they have a patent nostril and use the best side.
- Spray 5% lidocaine up the nostril and tell them to sniff. Give them a tissue and warn them that it is unpleasant and that their eyes will run. Sometimes patients in the head and neck clinic who are used to this procedure ask not to have the lidocaine spray.
- The nurse will have set up the scope for you. Don't do this alone—you won't know the sterilization and cross-infection rules.
- Check that the light source is working and try reading something on the side through the scope before you start to ensure that it is in focus and the lens piece is placed in such a way that up is up and down is down. Adjust if necessary.
- If you are lucky enough to have a camera and a display screen, check that these work. Most cameras are digital these days and photographs may be useful for writing case reports of unusual findings!
- Apply some water-based lubricant to the side of the tip of the scope.
- Slip the end of the scope over the nasal sill and run it along the floor of the nose at the base of the septum.
- You will pass over the soft palate, and by using the controller point the tip down as you go over the back of the palate.
- It is often helpful to ask the patient to swallow at this stage to clean mucus from the lens. You can also gently clean the lens by rubbing it on mucosa but you may make it bleed.
- You should be able to inspect the pharynx and larynx as far as the vocal cords in this way.
- If you ask the patient to say 'Eeeh', you will see the cords in function and can assess their symmetry of movement and see their surface.
- If they blow their cheeks out it can make it easier to assess the crevices, especially around the tongue base and valleculae.
- On the way out have a look at the nasopharynx around the opening of the Eustachian tubes and look at the upper surface of the soft palate and nose.

Taking dental impressions

If you are dentally qualified you will not need to read this section.

General points

- Ideally you should have a dental nurse with you.
- Position the patient sitting upright in a dental chair with head support so their mouth is just above elbow height.
- You will probably be using alginate (see p. 253).
- Find some impression trays and try them in first. Ensure that they can be seated over the teeth and extend back far enough.
- Check if there are any really loose teeth, crowns, or bridges. They could come out in the impression material, but it may help to coat them in white soft paraffin to stop it sticking.
- Remove any dentures, unless you are doing a special impression with the denture in, which is unlikely in OMFS.
- Has the patient had this done before? If so, did they have problems? Some patients just gag too much and are not really suitable for a novice.
- Load the tray with the impression material. It should be like mashed potato, not pureed potato, so it should not just flow out of the tray.
- For the upper impression seat it at the back first and then rock it so that it sits anteriorly also.
- Make sure that it is centrally positioned and lift up the lip and look at the soft palate. If it is running down the throat, scoop out the excess material with a finger but keep the tray in place with your other hand.
- Hold the tray firmly in place until the nurse tells you the material has set.
- Remove the tray by pulling sharply down. This is best done by tilting the tray so that the back (palatal area) comes away first. If it is difficult, try releasing around the edges.
- For the lower impression seat the tray at the back first (retromolar area) and ask the patient to lift up their tongue. You may need to pull the lower lip out of the way.
- Remove by lifting up sharply by the handle—again, a rotating motion to lift up the back first often works best.
- The patient will want to wash out their mouth and clean their face.
- The nurse will show you how the impressions must be cleaned and prepared before going to the labotatory.
- Fill in the laboratory work request card carefully, explaining exactly what you want. If there is any uncertainty go to the laboratory and talk to the technicians—it will save you time in the long run. It is also a good time to meet the laboratory staff and have a cup of coffee with them.

Cricothyroidotomy

General points

- You have probably completed an approved ATLS (or similar) course and understand the role of a cricothyroidotomy in emergency situations. However, such is the importance of this technique that we felt it would be worthwhile including a reminder section in this book.
- You may have only performed a cricothyroidotomy on a course, but unlike some of the other procedures trainees do on courses you must realize that a situation could arise where you are the only person available trained to do one and in such a case you must 'step up to the mark'.
- You can prepare for this in a number of ways.
  - First, read this section.
  - Secondly, think about doing cricothyroidotomies when you are in theatre with a senior. Palpate the landmarks, and run through with your senior about how you would do it.
  - Thirdly, if a tracheostomy is being done, try to make yourself available as they are a good time to discuss this procedure.
  - Finally, if you are called to see a patient with a potential emergency airway problem think about the worst-case scenario on your way there and re-read this chapter!
- When you arrive be aware that a tracheostomy is not an emergency procedure, and in almost every scenario a cricothyroidotomy is the life-saving procedure of choice. Do not assume that the anaesthetist or trauma leader knows how to do a 'crico'. Let them know you do!

The cricothyroidotomy

- Ideally the patient will be supine and motionless, but often they may be agitated and hypoxic.
- If you have time prepare some equipment such as a good light source, suction, oxygen, a cricothryroidotomy kit if possible and some oxygen, tubing, and tracheal dilators. Obviously if you have not got everything you might need but no time to wait, you will just have to get on with it.
- With your non-dominant hand hold the thyroid cartilage between your thumb and middle finger; your elbow is over the patient forehead. Using your index finger palpate the thyroid protuberance and follow it down to the criciothyroid membrane, which is not particularly soft. About a finger's breadth further south you will feel the cricoid cartilages as a hard raised ring; come back north again to the membrane and be decisive that this is the membrane. Mark it with a pen if you have time (Fig. 8.1).
- If the patient still conscious you may need to use some LA and skin cleanser.
- You can now do either a needle or a surgical cricothryroidotomy.
- A needle cricothryroidotomy will buy you about 30–40min. Push a criciothyroidotomy needle, if you have one, through the membrane, but if not use a large 14G venflon. A syringe on the needle can be used to confirm correct position. Air will be drawn back!

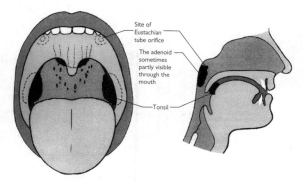

Site of
Eustachian
tube orifice

The adenoid
sometimes
partly visible
through the
mouth

Tonsil

Fig. 8.1 Oral cavity AP and oropharynx/nasopharynx lateral. Reproduced from Corbridge R, Steventon N *Oxford Handbook of ENT and Head and Neck Surgery*, p.185 (Oxford: 2010). With permission from Oxford University Press.

- Connect immediately to an oxygen source with a valve system to allow expiration, and put the oxygen on maximum flow. You now need to prepare for a definitive airway, and probably the best option still is to convert the needle cricothyroidotomy into a surgical cricothryroidotomy using the needle as a guide.
- The landmarks for a surgical cricothyroidotomy are the same as for a needle cricothyroidotomy, but you must make a horizontal incision through the skin overlying the membrane and then cut the membrane itself. There may be a lot of bleeding, but be bold and calm. Hold the thyroid cartilage firmly and make a 2cm incision through the skin and membrane. Then dilate with tracheal dilators (if available). Use these so that they spread the tissues in the long axis of the trachea and insert either a dedicated cricothyroidotomy tube, if you have one, or any tube you can find. Size 6 usually fits. Put the balloon up and connect to oxygen.
- Well done. You have just saved the patient's life!

Oral medicine

Common dental diseases

Dental caries

Dental caries is the result of acid-producing bacteria (*Streptococcus mutans* and others) creating a microenvironment, dental plaque, where sugar is metabolized and acid is a by-product. The acid demineralizes the tooth. The process is reversible when the pH rises and saliva, which is rich in Ca^{2+} ions, can reverse this demineralization. However, if demineralization predominates, cavitation will ensue. This will eventually lead to pulpal death, periapical infection, and subsequent abscess or chronic sinus formation. Early demineralization will be difficult to diagnose, and for the best results the tooth should be air dried and examined in good light. Bite wing radiographs are also helpful. Once a cavity has formed, it will need treatment either by filling or, if the hole is very large, by extraction.

Toothache

The pain of toothache comes either from the nerve endings within the pulp of the tooth (pulpal pain) or from the nerves in the periodontal membrane around the tooth (periodontal pain).

Pulpal pain

Tooth pulp does not contain any proprioceptors so pulpal pain is poorly localized.

Acute pulpitis can result from chemical, bacterial, thermal, or physical insults. The inflammation is either irreversible, which leads to pulp death, or reversible. Reversible pulpitis is usually a fleeting pain as a result of hot, cold, or sometimes sweet foods. It can be treated by dental restorations and dressings. Irreversible pulpitis is often of spontaneous onset and longer lasting. It requires RCT or extraction.

Another cause of pulpal pain is dentine/cemental sensitivity to heat, foods, and touching. This is usually due to exposed dentine and can be treated by sealing the exposed dentinal tubules with fluoride varnish (e.g. Duraphat) or regular use of desensitizing toothpastes.

Finally, cracked tooth syndrome is a toothache caused by biting and the name is self-explanatory. The dentist can often save the tooth if the crack is not too large.

Periapical pain

The periodontal membrane contains proprioceptors and so periodontitis is very well localized.

Periapical infection usually follows pulpal necrosis and can cause an acute apical periodiontits which is acutely painful. The tooth is very tender to tap—it is pushed out of the socket slightly so biting on it causes agony! The treatment is either extraction or RCT, or occasionally surgical drainage through the alveolar bone.

Acute apical periodontitis can also follow trauma and may resolve if the trauma is relieved.

Chronic periodontitis is usually associated with a draining abscess and may be asymptomatic.

Pericoronitis

This is inflammation of the flap of gum (operculum) over an erupting or impacted tooth, which is most commonly a lower wisdom tooth. Because the tooth cannot erupt normally, the gum cannot form a tight seal around the neck of the tooth, and bacteria and food debris accumulate under the gum flap causing local infection. This is often acute on chronic and anaerobic. The operculum swells and the condition may be worsened by the over-erupted opposing tooth (it has over-erupted because of the failure of the lower 8 to hold it back in occlusion) The initial treatment is an oral antibiotic such as metronidazole. Corsodyl® mouthwash may also be helpful. As an intermediary measure consider removal of the upper 8. Severe pericoronitis is an indication for removal of the lower 8 after the acute infection has settled.

Abnormalities of tooth structure

Dental enamel may appear pitted or grooved because of abnormalities of enamel matrix formation. This is termed hypoplasia. The enamel may be hypomineralized and initially appears opaque but tends to become discoloured with time. Causes can be congenital or acquired, and include drugs (fluoride), severe systemic diseases such as measles or rubella during development, and congenital causes including amelogenesis imperfecta and trisomy 21. Dentinogenesis imperfecta is more common and type I is associated with osteogenesis imperfecta. Staining of teeth can also be secondary to long-term tetracycline use (for acne) during tooth development.

Gingivitis

Gingivitis is literally inflammation of the gingivae or 'gums'. It appears as inflamed, red, and edematous gums which may bleed easily. Possible causes are as follows.

- A hormonal reaction in puberty and pregnancy.
- A reaction to drugs such as ciclosporin, nifedepine, and phenytoin.
- Virus, e.g primary herpetic gingivostomatitis.
- Bacteria, e.g. acute streptococcal gingivitis.
- It can also occur as part of other oral diseases such as oral lichen planus and pemphigoid, which is usually marginal.
- The most common cause is dental plaque, and gingivitis occurs wherever plaque accumulates. By definition, gingivitis is not a cause of alveolar bone loss or loss of attachment of the gum to the tooth except in acute ulcerative gingivitis (AUG), which is really a periodontal condition as bone loss is a feature.

Periodontitis

The periodontium includes those structures which support the teeth, the gums, periodontal membrane and alveolar bone. Periodontitis is a progression of gingivitis into the deeper tissues and is combination of loss of attachment of the periodontal membrane and resorption of the alveolar bone. Some individuals are more susceptible than others and may lose their teeth quite early as a result. It may be familial.

Necrotizing periodontal disease or AUG is a destructive acute condition caused by Gram-negative anaerobes. It leads to foul breath and rapid destruction of the periodontium. It may be a precursor to cancrum oris. It is treated by debridement, irrigation, chlorhexidine, and metronidazole (see p. 250).

Oral mucosal infections

In this section we cover some of the oral infections that are not covered elsewhere or are worthy of repetition.

Acute ulcerative gingivitis

- AUG is a rare destruction condition. It used to be called 'trench mouth' and is more common in run-down, debilitated, and HIV patients.
- It causes a foul smell, loss of the interdental papillae, and a metallic taste.
- It leaves craters where the papillae were, and in developing countries can proceed to cancrum oris.
- It is often confused with primary herpetic gingivostomatitis.
- Management includes debridement, irrigation, Corsodyl®, and metronidazole.

Candida

- *Candida* species are common oral commensals. The most important are *C.albicans* and *C.dublineisis*.
- Like all commensals they can cause disease if the immune system or local environment tips in their favour. This disease is called candidiasis.
- Candidiasis presents as sore areas, smooth patches, white patches (that can be rubbed off), or red patches.
- Management involves treating the cause as well as treating the candidiasis itself with antifungal therapy (such as oral fluconazole 50mg od for 7 days). Failure to treat the cause may lead to non-diagnosis of an important condition such as diabetes or HIV.

Acute candidiasis

- Acute pseudomembranous candidiasis (thrush) is the best known and occurs in the very young, the very old, the immunocompromised (especially cytotoxics, HIV, leukaemia, diabetes, etc.), and patients on long-term broad-spectrum antibiotics. The creamy film can be wiped off, leaving a red area underneath. The diagnosis is usually obvious, but if in doubt a sample can be sent to microbiology. Treat the cause where possible plus antifungal therapy as appropriate to the case, i.e. systemic fluconazole might be appropriate for the dangerously immunocompromised patient but might be over-treating an infant.
- Acute erythematous candidiasis occurs in patients taking broad-spectrum antibiotics or inhaled steroids (who fail to rinse their mouth out properly afterwards), or those with xerostomia or HIV. It presents as a red sore area(s), often in association with thrush. Treatment is as described for thrush.

Chronic candidiasis

- Chronic atrophic candidiasis occurs under dentures and presents as a red area under the fitting surface of the denture. The treatment is to clean the denture in a dilute solution of hypochlorite overnight and add miconazole gel to the surface of the dentures twice daily. Check if the patient is anaemic, diabetic, or immunocompromised if it persists.
- Angular chielitis is a mixed infection by staphylococci, β-haemolytic streptococci, and candida. The predisposing factors are also mixed and include poor dentures, anaemia, diabetes, and other immunocompromise. Treat the predisposing factors, and try miconazole cream which works on all three pathogens. If it persists, obtain a microbiology culture and ensure that you have not missed a predisposing factor.
- Median rhomboid glossitis causes a sore smooth area in the middle of the dorsum of the tongue. It is more common in smokers and those on inhaled steroids and with anaemia. Find the cause and treat as described above.
- Chronic hyperplastic candidiasis occurs just inside the corners of the mouth or on the dorsum of the tongue, mainly in heavy smokers. It may be pre-premalignant. Treat the underlying causes, as above, stop smoking, and give systemic antifungals. If it persists, surgical excision may be better. Do not discharge unless completely eradicated. Worthwhile biopsying to exclude underlying dysplasia.

Tuberculosis

- The most common presentation of TB in OMFS clinics is a neck lump, sometimes with systemic symptoms such as weight loss or night sweats. It is important to exclude lymphoma.
- Oral involvement can occur, especially with open pulmonary disease or coexisting HIV (may not be classical *Mycobacterium tuberculosis* in this case).
- The most common site is the posterior tongue.
- Diagnosis is by biopsy.

Syphilis

- Primary syphilis presents as a firm painless ulcerated chancre which is highly infectious and resolves after a couple of months.
- Secondary syphilis develops after 2–4 months as oral 'snail-track' ulcers, which are also highly contagious.
- Tertiary syphilis occurs after many years as gumma which are necrotic granulomata and are not infectious.
- It can also present as congenital syphilis with a saddle nose and abnormalities of tooth morphology (Hutchinson's incisors and mulberry molars).

Gonorrhea

- This is much more common than syphilis and leads to superficial ulcers of the oral cavity.

Oral ulceration

General but important points

- An ulcer is simply a breach in the oral epithelium with exposure of the underlying connective tissue.
- The list of causes of oral ulceration you will find in textbooks is almost limitless and confusing. In practice you will mainly see (in no particular order)
  - traumatic ulceration
  - recurrent aphthous ulceration
  - various autoimmune diseases
  - GI diseases
  - cancer and pre-cancerous lesions
  - ulcers induced by nicorandil or other drugs
  - infections, mainly viral ulceration.
- Biopsy is the best way to diagnose or to exclude cancer but is poor at diagnosing most other causes, e.g. other than malignancy, dysplasia, pemphigoid (maybe), pemphigus (possibly), or lichenoid, a biopsy may be reported as non-specific ulceration ± candida. So don't rely completely on biopsy. It is embarrassing when a patient has been followed up for months with a painful ulcer on the tongue which has been biopsied (non-specific ulceration) before someone notices that they are taking nicorandil!
- In the history note how long the ulcer has been present, any symptoms (especially otalgia), and if single or multiple, recurrent, persistent. Was it accompanied by systemic illness?
- In the systems enquiry look for bowel disease, ulcers elsewhere, especially genitalia and anus, eye disease, anaemia, weight loss, fatigue, skin rashes.
- Record risk factors such as smoking, especially if recently stopped, alcohol use, occupation, ethnic origin, social history.
- In previous medical history look for drugs, GI diseases, anaemia, eye disease, dermatological disease.
- In examination check cervical nodes and record site and size of all oral lesions (📖 see p. 34). Feel the ulcer—is it surrounded by hardness? This induration may be a sign of malignancy.
- Bilateral and recurrent lesions are rarely malignant.
- If you think that the ulcer is caused by a sharp tooth or loose denture flange, treat the cause immediately and arrange follow-up 2 weeks later—no longer or you may be caught out.
- Any ulcer present for more than 3 weeks without obvious cause must be biopsied immediately, but first exclude nicorandil-induced ulceration, rubbing denture flanges, sharp teeth, etc.

Recurrent aphthous stomatitis (RAS)

- This is common condition which affects about 25% of the population at some time in their life. It usually starts in young age and may burn out in adulthood. Most GPs manage the condition without referring the patient to hospital, some do not, and some cases are more severe.

- There are many theories about RAS, but in reality it is an incurable idiopathic condition. Most patients manage to live with it, but like all conditions there are extreme variants.
- There are three subtypes of RAS:
  - In minor aphthous stomatitis the ulcers are <5mm in size. Usually one to five occur on the non-keratinized mucosa and heal in 1–2 weeks without scarring. This is the most common type.
  - In major aphthous stomatitis the ulcers are larger, less numerous, more painful, last longer, and may occur on the keratinized mucosa. They eventually heal with scarring.
  - In herpetiform aphthous stomatitis (nothing to do with herpes!) the ulcers are small and numerous. They may coalesce but don't scar. This is the rarest type.
- When taking a history ask about a prodromal phase of itching/altered sensation in the mucosa followed by recurrent painful ulcers.
- Consider if there could be an underlying GI disease or a haematinic deficiency. Ask about genital ulcers (Behçet's syndrome) or eye symptoms (pemphigoid).
- If the GP has not already done so, check the haematinics (vitamin B_{12}, folate and ferritin) and zinc.
- Once you have excluded everything else and the history is typical, spend some time informing patient about the condition:
- It will become worse with stress. It may be related to menstrual cycle and may be familial. Even those without haematinic deficiency may recover on multivitamins, especially vitamin B_{12} and zinc. Others use Corsodyl® to prevent bacterial super-infection. Some use tetracycline mouthwash. Topical local anaesthetic agents (betametasone) have no therapeutic benefit but may help if pain is very severe. Topical steroids (hydrocortisone 2.5mg pellets, betametasone mouthwash (500mcg in 20ml H_2O used for 1–2min tds when severe and then spat out) or even systemic steroids help.

Do not arrange a follow-up, unless a senior tells you otherwise. Most clinics refer back to GP. If further help is needed, an oral medicine referral might be more appropriate.

A word about nicorandil

- Nicorandil is a vasodilatory drug used to treat ischaemic heart disease.
- It can cause ulceration anywhere along the GI tract, and cases of small bowel perforation and anal ulceration have been described as well as oral ulceration.
- The oral ulcers are very painful and start months after the drug has been started. They will resolve a couple of months after the drug has been stopped.
- The biopsy will show non-specific inflammation and make the ulcer even more painful, and it will heal very slowly.
- The diagnosis is often slow, and patients may have had many months of painful oral ulceration.
- Ask the patient's GP or cardiologist to stop the drug if possible and review the patient.

Blistering diseases

General points
- These are autoimmune blistering mucocutaneous diseases.
- They can be divided into those that cause intra-epithelial blisters (pemphigus) and those that cause sub-epithelial blisters (pemphigoid).
- They are uncommon conditions, but the oral features may appear early in the course of the disease and hence it may be you who makes the diagnosis.
- The sub-epithelial blistering diseases include:
  - pemphigoid
  - dermatitis herpetiformis
  - erythema multiforme
  - toxic epidermal necrolysis.

Mucous membrane pemphigoid
- This is the most common of the sub-epithelial blistering conditions.
- It affects the mucous membranes and/or the skin.
- Antibodies are directed against the basement membrane.
- There is a mainly oral variant which is associated with anti-integrin antibodies.
- The mainly ocular variant may also affect the mouth and is associated with anti-epiligrin antibodies.
- The oral lesions mainly affect the gingivae and palate, and constitute blisters which may be tense and blood-filled or rupture and become ulcers.
- The other feature is patchy desquamative gingivitis. This may be the sole feature and can be mistaken for periodontal disease.
- Untreated ocular involvement can lead to blindness.
- Laryngeal scarring can lead to stenosis.
- Diagnosis is by biopsy of perilesional tissue and needs specialized histological and immunostaining assessment. It is also important to place the biopsy in a special transport medium (Michel's medium).
- Indirect immunofluorescence (blood test) is often negative.
- Management depends on severity, but steroids and tacrolimus are the mainstay.
- Specialist management and liaison with the dermatologist may be necessary, and other drugs including dapsone and azathioprine may be required.

Erythema multiforme (EM)
- This is an acute condition which may recur.
- It is an autoimmune disease which is triggered by factors such as herpes simplex and drugs (including penicillins and some anaesthetic agents).
- It is more common in young males.
- The skin lesions may be symmetrical macules or ring-shaped target lesions on the extremities.
- Oral lesions include ulceration and crusting of the lips with blisters and ulcers elsewhere in the mouth. They may recur in about 25%.

- Periodicity may vary from weeks to years. Attacks last for 1–3 weeks.
- The disease usually burns out after about five or six attacks.
- There is no diagnostic test for EM but it can be helpful to take serum samples for HSV. Biopsy may support the clinical diagnosis but is not in itself diagnostic.
- There is no specific treatment for EM.
- Management may include antiviral therapy and topical or systemic corticosteroids, but this is controversial.
- Major EM, Stevens–Johnson syndrome may require admission for rehydration and analgesia.
- Toxic epidermal necrolysis is a more severe form of this condition, with skin detachment all over the body. It is life threatening.

Pemphigus

- Pemphigus refers to a group of life threatening intra-epithelial blistering diseases.
- Because the blisters are intra-epithelial, they rupture more easily and lead to severe ulceration. Slight rubbing of the skin/mucosa leads to Nikolsky's sign—exfoliation of the outermost layer. This sign is also seen in toxic epidermal necrolysis, but not in pemphigoid.
- Pemphigus can lead to fluid loss, electrolyte imbalance, scarring and its complications, deformity, dysfunction of essential processes such as eating, breathing, and digestion, and ultimately, if untreated, death.
- Pemphigus vulgaris is the most severe form and leads not only to skin ulceration but also to blisters and ulcers of any or all of the following: mouth, nose, oesophagus, anus, larynx, rectum, conjunctiva, and genitalia.
- The first lesions to present may be on the scalp and in the mouth.
- Diagnosis is same as pemphigoid, but serum titres of antibody may help to guide treatment as it corresponds to the disease severity.
- Patients must be referred to chest physician, GI physician, dermatologist, and ophthalmic surgeon.
- Management usually involves oral prednisolone and other immuno-suppressants.
- Approximately 75% of patients can discontinue therapy after 10 years, but the oral lesions tend to be recalcitrant.

Bullous lichen planus

- This is a rare variant of a fairly common mucocutaneous autoimmune disorder which, when the blisters break, can leave sub-epithelial ulcers (see p. 222).

White, red, and pigmented lesions

White lesions

General points

- Some white patches in the mouth can be wiped off (causes include thrush, plaque/food debris, or a collapsed blister or a burn) but others cannot.
- Most white patches in the mouth which cannot be wiped off are caused by an increase in the amount of keratin. Keratin is a protein which absorbs water and when it reaches a certain thickness appears white (see how white your calluses are when you have been in the swimming pool).
- There are may causes of an increase in keratin (hyperkeratosis)—physiological response to a stimulus, pathological process, or neo-plastic effect. Causes include:
  - lichen planus
  - leukoplakia
  - cancer
  - trauma
  - white spongy naevus.
- Leukoplakia, defined as a white patch of unknown cause which cannot be classified into any other diagnosis, can be dysplastic and pre-malignant (especially the heterogenous forms).

Lichen planus (LP)

- Oral LP is probably one of the most common diseases of the oral mucosa that you will see in OMFS clinics.
- LP affects ~2% of people at some time in their life. Half of those with skin lesions also have oral lesions, but a quarter of cases have oral lesions only.
- LP is an autoimmune incurable condition treated mainly by topical steroids if symptomatic. These include betamethasone mouthwash (500mcg in 20ml H_2O used for 1–2min tds when severe and then spat out) or a beclometasone inhaler.
- Oral LP is invariably bilateral and may cause desquamative gingivitis, striations, papules, plaques, bullae, erosions, atrophic areas, or ulcers.
- The skin lesions affect the flexor surfaces of the arms and the tibial region of the legs with purple papules covered in tiny white striae.
- Diagnosis is supported by histology, but note that a lichenoid reaction looks the same histologically. Lichenoid reaction is usually unilateral and most commonly related to an amalgam filling. It may also be caused by a change in toothpaste.

Friction-induced hyperkeratosis

- An increase in keratin will occur as a physiological response to friction—look at the soles of your feet!
- It is most common on the buccal mucosa along the occlusal line, when it is called linea alba.
- It also occurs on the alveolus where teeth have been lost and the opposing tooth is rubbing food against the gum.

- It can occur on the lips or the tip of the tongue, usually as a result of habitual biting or rubbing.
- The diagnosis is usually clear, but histology will exclude other causes such as dysplasia and malignancy.

Red lesions

- Oral lesions are red because either there is more blood in the mucosa than normal (inflammation, vascular lesion) or the mucosa is thinner than normal (erosion, atrophy, neoplasia).
- Erythroplakia is a pre-malignant condition which is a red patch not caused by anything else—it should be biopsied. Histology may show dysplasia.
- Generally speaking, red patches need much closer attention than white patches, and biopsy is more likely to be helpful
- Speckled leukoplakia is a sinister lesion which is invariably either premalignant or malignant and is discussed in the next section (see p. 224).

Pigmented lesions

- In managing oral pigmentation it is valuable to subdivide the lesions into localized and multiple or generalized.
- Localized causes include:
  - amalgam tattoo
  - Kaposi's sarcoma
  - melanoma
  - melanotic macule (melanosis—may be trauma related)
  - naevus
  - ephelis (freckle)
  - black hairy tongue;
- Multiple or generalized causes include:
  - racial pigmentation
  - drugs
    — ACTH
    — amiodarone and others
  - Endocrine
    — Addison's disease
    — Albright's syndrome
    — Nelson's syndrome
    — pregnancy (not a disease!)
  - Peutz–Jeghers syndrome
- If you are in doubt and the lesion is solitary, take an excisional biopsy. If it is multiple, look at drugs—everything else is very rare.

Oral cancer

General points

- SCC is the most common cancer of the oral cavity and is the sixth most common cancer worldwide. It is the most common cancer in the Indian subcontinent (because of betel nut chewing).
- It is caused mainly by alcohol, tobacco, HPV16, and betel nut.
- Oral cancer in young people seems to be increasing—more than six oral sex partners significantly increases risk.[1]
- The mainstay of treatment is still surgery.
- Early diagnosis is critical to improving survival. Metastasis to the neck is the single most important prognostic indicator, and when present reduces the chances of survival by 50%.
- Most oral cancer referrals for oral lesions come from dentists, while most oral cancer presentations with nodal metastasis to the neck come from GPs.
- Other cances types can be found in the oral cavity. There is an extensive list including salivary gland tumours, metastases, melanoma, sarcomas, and haematological malignancies. These will not be discussed further here.

Premalignant conditions

- Leuoplakia (especially heterogenous), erythroplakia, and speckled leukoplakia are all potentially pre-malignant and where possible should be excised completely. These patients need close monitoring as well as stopping all risk habits such as betel nut chewing, smoking, etc.
- Oral submucous fibrosis (again related to betel nut chewing) and oral lichen planus (particularly the atrophic form, although some authorities question this) may undergo malignant transformation and should be monitored.
- Sideropenic dysphagia, Fanconi's anaemia, and syphilis are also significant risk factors. The first two require very close observation, while syphilis requires antibiotics.

Diagnosis

- SCC of the oral cavity presents as a lump, ulcer, white patch, or red patch, or a mixture of all these. Diagnosis is by biopsy.
- Cancers of the oropharynx may be more difficult to diagnose. Sometimes the presenting features are neck lumps, otalgia, odinophagia, dysphagia, or a hoarse voice, and require MRI, PET-CT, FNAC, and EUA biopsy.
- Never dismiss sudden onset of otalgia in an adult—it can be the first sign of a tongue cancer (with lingual nerve involvement) or oropharyngeal cancer.

Staging

- Oral and oropharyngeal cancer is staged using the TNM system (Table 9.1) and can be clinical, radiological, or pathological.

1 D'Souza G, Kreimer AR, Viscidi R, *et al.* (2007). *New England Journal of Medicine* **356**: 1944–56.

Table 9.1 The TNM classification

T	Primary tumour	N	Cervical nodes
T1	<2cm diameter	**N0**	No nodes
T2	2–4cm diameter	**N1**	Single node <3cm
T3	>4cm diameter	**N2**	Single 3–6cm node (N2a), multiple nodes (N2b), or contralateral nodes (N2c)
T4	Massive, invading other structures	**N3**	Node >6cm
		M	Distant metastases
		M0	Absent
		M1	Present

Reproduced from Mitchell L, Mitchell D. *Oxford Handbook of Clinical Dentistry*, p.416 (Oxford: 2009). With permission from Oxford University Press

Principles of treatment

- Decision-making in oral cancer is an MDT process.
- The single most important question is: Is the disease curable?
- The second most important question is: What are the curative options and what are the complications/side effects of these options?
- The third question is related to the management of the neck. Does this need treating? Are there metastases already or does the primary tumour have a high risk of occult metastasis? A tumour depth >4mm is associated with a much greater risk of neck metastasis.
- It is then down to the patient and the MDT to decide together. Some patients may choose non-curative (but life-extending) treatments because the side effects of curative (but not guaranteed) treatment are too unpleasant.
- Surgical excision with reconstruction and adjuvant radiotherapy ± chemotherapy is the mainstay of most oral cancer treatment.
- Oropharyngeal cancers are usually treated with organ-preserving radiotherapy (in combination with chemotherapy). In these cases surgery is reserved for residual or recurrent disease.
- About 2% of major head and neck cancer patients who undergo surgery die within 30 days.
- About 60% have some complication including myocardial infarction, cerebrovascular accident, pneumonia, neck infection, flap failure, skin graft failure, and countless others.
- The side effects of radiotherapy include osteoradionecrosis, mucositis, skin ulceration, dysphagia, xerostomia, haematological malignancy, etc.

Oral manifestations of systemic diseases

HIV

- This immunodeficiency state causes oral conditions in 75% of cases but none are diagnostic.
- Group I conditions are strongly associated with HIV infection:
  - candidiasis, especially thrush
  - hairy leukoplakia—EBV-related bilateral white corrugated lesions of tongue
  - HIV gingivitis—more severe than one would otherwise expect for the general state of the mouth
  - AUG
  - Kaposi's sarcoma—this requires biopsy and often presents as a purple lump on the palate
  - non-Hodgkin's lymphoma (e.g. Burkitt's lymphoma) is much more common in HIV patients.
- Group II conditions are less strongly associated:
  - atypical oropharyngeal ulceration.
  - idiopathic thrombocytopenic purpura
  - salivary gland disease.
- Group III conditions are possibly associated:
  - bacterial and fungal infections
  - cat scratch disease (toxoplasmosis)
  - SCC
  - others.
- Clinically the most important thing to know is that if you see any group I conditions you must consider HIV. The most common ones you will actually spot in OMFS clinics are hairy leukoplakia and thrush.

GI disease

- Coeliac disease may cause oral ulceration, which may be the presenting symptom in adults
- Ulcerative colitis can cause ulcers which look just like aphthous ulcers.
- Crohn's disease can cause swelling of the oral mucosa and lips and cause linear ulcers or cobblestone appearance of the mucosa.
- Orofacial granulomatosis is indistinguishable from oral manifestations of Crohn's disease, and is probably a hypersensitivity reaction to some foodstuffs such as benzoates and cinnaminides.

Haematological disease

- Deficiencies of iron, vitamin B_{12}, and folate can all cause recurrent aphthous stomatitis.
- Iron-deficiency anaemia can also cause atrophic glossitis, angular cheilitis, oral candidiasis, and a sore or burning tongue or mouth.
- Leukaemia can cause oral diseases in many ways. They may present with immunocompromise-induced oral infections.

- Leukaemia may also present as a deposit in the gingiva which bleeds easily. Occasionally bleeding gums in children is the first presentation of leukaemia.
- The chemotherapy drugs used in the treatment of leukaemias are themselves immunosuppressants and may lead to oral infection and bleeding.
- IV bisphosphonates, such as alendronate, are commonly used in multiple myeloma and other cancers which have bony metastases (such as advanced breast and prostate cancer). They can cause bisphosphonate-related osteonecrosis of the jaws (BRONJ), an unpleasant condition resulting in destruction of the jaw bones, often secondary to dental extractions or ulceration of the gum. BRONJ is more common in the mandible than in the maxilla (possibly because of poorer blood supply).

Endocrine disease

- Poorly controlled diabetes can cause all the effects of immuno-compromise including severe dento-cervical abscesses, periodontitis, sialosis (bilateral soft enlargement of the parotid glands), burning mouth, and thrush.
- Hyperparathyroidism can lead to destructive radiolucent lesions within the jaws which are indistinguishable from giant cell granulomas.
- Acromegaly can cause enlargement of the lips, tongue, and mandible, with spacing of the teeth. A changing occlusion in an adult ('my teeth don't meet, doctor') with a prognathic mandible is a giveaway for this condition and should prompt you to check growth hormone levels.

Miscellaneous oral conditions

Jaw cysts

- Cysts are more common in the jaws than in any other bones of the body mainly because of the epithelial remnants of tooth development.
- The most common jaw cyst is the radicular cyst, or inflammatory dental cyst, which develops around the root apex as a result of infection. It can persist after the tooth is extracted, when it is called a residual cyst. If untreated it will continue to grow and resorb bone (but rarely results in root resorption). It is treated by enucleation.
- Dentigerous cysts result from degeneration of the follicle around the crown of a permanent tooth. They will also resorb bone and occasionally roots. Most commonly occur around impacted upper canines and lower 8s, and cystic change may be an indication for these teeth to be removed.
- Keratocysts, or keratocystic odontogenic tumours, are derived from remnants of the dental lamina and are problematic as they can grow very large, resorb bone and teeth, and may recur after simple enucleation because of the presence of daughter cysts within the capsule. They may be unilocular or multilocular, and are most common in the posterior mandible but can occur anywhere in the jaws. After enucleation, the surrounding bone is often burred away, or liquid nitrogen can be placed. Historically Carnoy's solution was used, but this is now difficult to obtain.
- There are a number of pseudocysts, such as solitary bone cyst and aneurysmal bone cyst. Both are treated by opening the cyst and cleaning out the contents.
- Ameloblastomas are benign tumours of the jaw which can present as cystic lesions on radiographs. They should be diagnosed by open biopsy before definitive treatment is planned. Although technically benign, they have a high propensity for recurrence and can be locally destructive. They can be likened to BCCs of the bone. They can behave like malignant tumours if and when they escape from the bone into the soft tissue.

Tongue tie

- It is not uncommon for children, accompanied by their anxious parents, to be referred to OMFS clinics with a tongue tie.
- The best option is probably to ask a paediatric SALT if they think a lingual frenectomy could be beneficial and act on that basis.
- Many children have very normal speech and swallowing with a tied tongue, and many children with speech anomalies do not have a tongue tie, but all children are different and it's a potential mine field.
- What you can't do with a tongue tie is French kiss, and some teenagers come for the snip! The judgement is pretty much up to you and/or your seniors.

Burning mouth syndrome

- A range of terms are used to describe strange sensations in the mouth with no obvious organic cause. They include oral dys-aesthesia, burning mouth syndrome, and burning tongue.
- They are all more common in post-menopausal women and may be related to low oestrogen.
- Diagnosis is only by exclusion. Occasionally (and with great relief) you will find a case of oral lichen planus, which is a great deal easier to treat than burning mouth syndrome!
- Take a full history. Is it worse in the morning, worse at the back of the throat, and associated with recent weight gain or dyspepsia and hoarse voice in the morning? If so, consider acid regurgitation, do a nasendoscopy looking for Renke's oedema, and start a PPI such as omeprazole
- Perhaps the symptoms began after changing or starting a new medication. Look up the side effects of the drug in the *British National Formulary*, stop or change—discuss with GP.
- Have they changed their toothpaste lately? Try changing back.
- Could they be anaemic? Are they vegetarian or vegan? Has there been a change of bowel habit, fatigue, etc?
- Is it worse with tomatoes or spicy food? This classically occurs with oral lichen planus.
- Examine the mouth fully and biopsy anything that looks abnormal.
- Check haematinics (vitamin B_{12}, folate, ferritin), fasting glucose, and zinc.
- If all the above are normal, you are left with the idiopathic diagnosis. Try multivitamins A–Z and review after 6 months.
- If they return and the symptoms are no better and no other disease/cause has presented itself, you may consider prescribing antidepressants.
- Discharge to GP. If further advice is needed, suggest specialist oral medicine.

Osteoradionecrosis of the jaws

- This is a side effect of radiotherapy to the jaws. It is more common if the patient is exposed to >60Gy and is more common in the mandible.
- It leads to bone death and often secondary infection of the overlying mucosa and to some extent the dead bone.
- Tooth extraction is often a precipitating event.
- It is painful and can result in pathological fracture.
- It may require resection and reconstruction.
- It differs from BRONJ in a number of ways, but in terms of treatment it is easier as it is more localized. However, radiotherapy to the neck and skin can cause problems if reconstructive surgery is planned, e.g. athermoma of the carotid tree can complicate free tissue transfer (increased risk of wound breakdown etc.).

Emergencies

The compromised airway

General points

- This is possibly the most important section in this book.
- It is written on assumption that you have ATLS training (or equivalent). We will not repeat basic facts, but give a gentle reminder that a tracheostomy is not an option in an emergency situation and you should be prepared to undertake a cricothyroidotomy from day one of an OMFS job.
- Read the section on cricothyrodoidotomy (◻ see p. 208) and get into the habit when you are in theatre of examining the patient's neck and asking yourself: 'Where is the criciothyroid membrane?'
- In OMFS you will encounter compromised airways in the following situations:
  - trauma
  - abscesses
  - tumour obstruction
  - postoperatively
    — unexpected bleeding and swelling
    — tracheostomy complications (◻ see p. 234).

The trauma patient

- ATLS rules apply.
- Trauma patients most commonly have airway problems because the fractured facial bones are posteriorly displaced, or there is bleeding into the pharynx, or there is a laryngeal injury.
- If possible, sit the patient up, lean them forwards, and suck out the mouth.
- Be prepared to physically pull fractured bones and the tongue forward to clear the obstructed airway.
- If you cannot do this because of the need for C-spine immobilization and clearance, you could log roll patient 180° on a stretcher so that they are facing the floor as a temporary measure until senior help arrives.
- If that is not an option, rapid sequence intubation is required and the trauma team leader should request this while you do what you can to help with suction and manipulation of fragments as above.

The postoperative patient

- This is more likely in orthognathic, FOM, and oncology surgery.
- Consider if removal of sutures and/or evacuation of a clot might help.
- 'Sit them up, give oxygen, suck out mouth and nose' should be the advice that you give over the phone whilst you are making your way briskly to the ward.
- Postoperative patients may be difficult intubations so the need for cricothyroidotomy is more likely.
- Get anaesthetic help early.

The abscess patient

- In these cases airway obstruction can be very sudden and is usually due to laryngeal oedema. The key to avoiding disasters is to spot the warning red flags and act quickly.
- You must never be left alone with these patients—get help.
- Patients die first from airway obstruction, so the priority is to secure the airway, not an immediate incision and drainage.
- Danger signs:
  - 'hot potato' voice
  - refusal to lie back
  - drooling of saliva
  - tachycardia
  - distressed
  - shortness of breath, tachypnoea, and falling oxygen saturation are **very** late signs.
- You must:
  - get anaesthetist **now**
  - give oxygen, get IV access
  - call for senior OMFS help.
- Management will depend to some extent on the anaesthetist's experience.
- If the anaesthetist is suitably trained they may wish to do an awake fibreoptic naso-endotracheal intubation, usually with needle crico-thyroidotomy *in situ*.
- If the anaesthetist is not trained in awake fibreoptic intubation and there is insufficient time to wait for someone who is, you must do something immediately. This probably means a cricothyroidotomy. If the anaesthetist attempts normal intubation, ensure that either the criciothyroid membrane is marked with permanent ink or, even better, you have inserted a needle cricothyroidotomy—this will buy you some time if the airway is lost and acts as a guide for surgical crico-thyroidotomy.
- You may not have time to wait until you get to theatre to do this.
- Use IV antibiotics, fluids, and dexamethasone by all means, but do not allow this to delay the securing of a definitive airway.
- Don't get bogged down with definitions like 'Ludwig's angina'. What matters to your patient right now is securing their airway.

The cancer patient

Patients with advanced tumours around the glottis and tongue base can present with acute loss of airway and require emergency crico-thyroidotomy or urgent tracheostomy. They may also have sudden bleeding (due to meta-static disease around the great vessels) which can cause rapid neck swelling and airway obstruction.

Tracheostomy tube problems

General points

- You need to be familiar with tracheostomy tubes and how they work (Figs 10.1 and 10.2).
- www.tracheostomy.org.uk is an excellent site for anyone who has anything to do with tracheostomies, and we advise you to look at this site now.
- It is important to appreciate that although tracheostomy tubes are designed to help with ventilation they can also be a source of obstruction.
- The most common problems you will have with tracheostomy tubes are blockage, displacement, and bleeding around them.

Blocked tracheostomy tubes

- If a patient is completely dependent on the tracheostomy tube for ventilation then a blockage is immediately life threatening. You must remove the inner tube if there is one, suction the outer tube, let the cuff down and give high flow oxygen. While doing this ask someone else (e.g. ward nurse) to call the crash team or at the very least to fast bleep the on call anaesthetist.
- If that still doesn't help, then you need to either remove the tube completely or if you have time and the ability, change it over a boogie.
- If you don't know how to change a tracheostomy tube and you do not have time to wait for someone else to arrive, take the tube out and see what happens. This often solves the problem but if not you must get an airway by some other means as quickly as possible. This may mean using a bag-valve-mask, laryngeal mask or intubation or even cricothyroidotomy. Unless you are experienced do NOT go exploring the neck with tracheal dilators in hope of finding the tracheal stoma. It is unlikely that you will find it and you are wasting precious time.
- If the patient is 'breathing around' a blocked tracheostomy tube, they may be struggling to breath but you have a bit more time to remove the inner tube, and to clean and suction. Let the cuff down and give oxygen as outlined above. Call for senior help quickly if no rapid improvement with these measures: e.g the diagnosis could be wrong and there may be need to have a look down the tube with a nasendoscope.

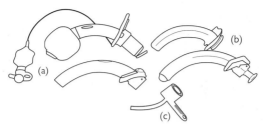

Fig. 10.1 Diagrams of tracheostomy tubes: (a) cuffed fenestrated tube; (b) non-cuffed non-fenestrated tube; (c) paediatric tube. Reproduced from Corbridge R, Steventon N. *Oxford Handbook of ENT and Head and Neck Surgery*, p.241 (Oxford: 2010). With permission from Oxford University Press.

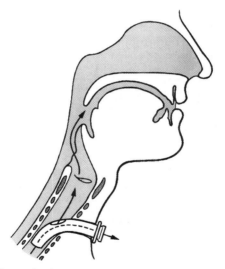

Fig. 10.2 Diagram of tracheostomy tube position (note fenestration). Reproduced from Corbridge R, Steventon N. *Oxford Handbook of ENT and Head and Neck Surgery*, p.241 (Oxford: 2010). With permission from Oxford University Press.

Displaced tubes
- If the tube is displaced within the first few days of placement the tract will rapidly close and re-insertion of tube will be near impossible except under controlled conditions.
- Therefore if you cannot see the tracheal stoma clearly (unless a Bjork flap has been used, this is unlikely) do not waste time trying to do the impossible, but get an airway by any other means. Use bag–valve–mask for the time being until the anaesthetist arrives. They will then consider intubation. You will still be of use because the anaesthetist will want to know what surgery has been done etc. We advocate the use of silk stay sutures placed at the time of tracheostomy to facilitate tube re-insertion. These simple sutures help to bring the tracheostomy stoma towards the skin and can greatly facilitate this manoeuvre.
- If bag–valve–mask ventilation is not successful, the anaesthetist has not arrived yet, and you are not trained to intubate, proceed immediately to cricothyroidotomy. Likewise if intubation is unsuccessful.
- When you are ventilating a patient with bag–valve–mask you may need to occlude the neck wound to obtain better ventilation, but don't think that if the air comes out it will be easy to get tube back in!

Bleeding around tracheostomy tubes
- Massive bleeding around the tube warrants the usual resuscitation steps and immediate return to theatre. Don't forget to inflate the cuff to protect the airway. Place two large-bore cannulae, cross-match 4 units, and tell your senior that the patient is on their way to theatre.
- Management of lesser bleeding may be more open to interpretation and discussion, so you should do the basics (get lines in, inflate cuff, cross-match, etc.) but call your senior before you arrange to return to theatre.
- Recent guidelines suggest that if the bleeding occurs >72 hours after placement of the tracheostomy tube the patient should return to theatre for endoscopic examination of the trachea to exclude inominate artery fistula.
- Inominate artery fistula can present with a smallish herald bleed followed by catastrophic and usually fatal bleeding.
- The other more common source of bleeding around tracheostomy tubes which have been in for a few days is the granulation tissue which forms around the tube and which bleeds easily. It is usually treated by packing some ribbon gauze around the tube and correcting any coagulopathies if appropriate.

Massive bleeding from the face and mouth

General points
The most common causes you will encounter are:
- facial fractures
- nosebleed not associated with facial fractures
- facial and oral lacerations.

Bleeding from facial fractures
- If safe to do so, sit the patient up and allow them to lean forward.
- Get a good light source and suction out mouth and anterior nose.
- Try to find the source of bleeding.
- Bleeding from midface (📖 see also pp. 74, 198).
  - Pass a Foley catheter along the nasal floor so that the balloon is just beyond the posterior nasal aperture and inflate balloon, both sides.
  - Pull the inflated balloons against theposterior nasal aperture and then pack the nasal cavity with nasal tampons, both sides.
  - Use a disposable drain clamp to secure the Foley catheters and maintain pressure.
  - Now try to impact the maxilla vertically by placing a bite block between the teeth.
- Bleeding from the mandible.
  - Try to reduce the fragments and compress across the fractures.
  - This may need LA and bridle wires (📖 see pp. 190, 201).
  - Beware of bleeding into the FOM which can posteriorly displace the tongue and obstruct the airway perhaps several hours later on the ward in the middle of night, so look for and manage it sooner rather than later.
- Bleeding from pan-facial fractures.
  - If both jaws are fractured it can be more difficult to control bleeding as the mandible will not compress the maxilla.
  - Place Foley catheters and pack the nose as before, reduce mandible fractures, and bridle wire if possible, but you may need to get the patient intubated and go to theatre immediately.
  - Intubation is usually via an oral endotracheal tube, but in theatre the team may need to consider tracheostomy or submental intubation to allow fixation of the mandible.

Bleeding from facial laceration
- Usually from facial, superficial temporal, or supra-orbital arteries.
- Stay calm and apply pressure with a carefully placed fresh gauze swab.
- Check observations and past medical history.
- Resuscitate and if past medical history dictates manage accordingly. For example, is the patient anticoagulated?
- Clean the area with sterile saline ± suction and apply pressure directly to the bleeding point. Examine the wound.
- Is there a facial nerve injury? Check this before you give any LA.

- Once you have done this, give LA around the wound. Sometimes this measure alone is enough to stop the bleeding because of the vaso-constriction properties of adrenaline in the LA cartridge.
- Only clip and tie the artery if you can see it clearly. You need to tie both ends of the vessel.
- Bipolar diathermy must be used with similar caution. Do not diathermy the facial nerve!
- If you are not happy to do this, clean the wound and apply pressure whilst you are waiting for senior help to arrive.
- The key to success is applying pressure directly to the bleeding point and not in a vague area through five already blood-soaked gauze swabs!

Nosebleed not associated with facial fractures

- Epistaxis is often idiopathic and spontaneous, but exacerbating medical problems include:
  - anticoagulation/coagulopathy
  - hypertension
  - hereditary haemorrhagic telangiectasia.
- Sit patient forward and pinch nostrils.
- Meanwhile resuscitate; two large-bore cannulae, G&S, coagulation screen, FBC including platelet count, and monitor response to resuscitation.
- If this doesn't work, you will need to pass nasal tampons down both sides of the nose (see p. 198).
- If this doesn't work, take the tampons out, pass Foley catheters (see p. 198), and then put new tampons in.
- Do not attempt nasal cautery unless you are trained to do so.
- If the bleeding persists despite the Foley catheters and tampons, get 4 units cross-matched urgently and increase fluid resuscitation. Chase the coagulation screen and obtain senior advice. Consider interventional radiology or endoscopic surgery (usually from ENT).
- The most common error in epistaxis is failure to appreciate the severity of blood loss and a failure to resuscitate the patient adequately.

Massive bleeding from the neck

General points

- In this section we will not discuss the subtleties of all penetrating neck injuries (📖 see p. 82), but only those with major bleeding.
- Usually one of two scenarios:
  - penetrating injury, usually stabbing
  - carotid blow-out.

Penetrating neck injuries

- ATLS all the way. Patients with neck stabbings can die from A, B, C, or even D if the spinal cord is hit, so don't go straight to C.
- Of special note.
  - Make sure you have the trauma team with you and work together as a team.
  - Get a definitive airway and be aware risk of lung injury at the B stage.
  - At C apply pressure to the bleeding site if possible. Get two large-bore cannulae in and request cross-match. Resuscitate and monitor—ideally this should be being done by a member of the team as the airway is being secured.
  - Your senior should be called.
- Resuscitate and if possible stabilize the patient, but what saves life is stopping the bleeding which means getting to theatre immediately.
- Don't delay this by sending patient to exsanguinate in a CT scanner!
- It can be helpful at stressful times like massive neck bleeds to have some classifications to hand for reminders, so here's one.
- The neck can be divided into three zones.
  - Zone I is base of neck—special risk of great vessel, lung, oesophagus, trachea, and brachial plexus injures.
  - Zone II is mid-neck—injuries to carotid, jugular, pharynx, larynx, and spinal cord, but less likely to be missed as easy to inspect.
  - Zone III is between angle of mandible and skull base—parotid glands, pharynx, spinal cord, and cranial nerves at risk. Difficult to inspect and access surgically.
- Do not be fooled by the neck bleed which stops and the patient becomes haemodynamically stable. It must be explored.

Carotid blow-out

- This is a horrendous situation to be in for everyone, so you will have to rise to the challenge. However, reading this section and your previous experience of ATLS should prepare you in some part.
- Carotid blow-out usually affects postoperative patients after resection with neck dissections, especially post-radiotherapy salvage surgery for recurrent disease.
- More likely if there has been some breakdown of the neck wound.
- May be preceded by a herald bleed. That is a lesson best learned in this section rather than at a morbidity and mortality (M&M) meeting.
- If you make diagnosis at herald bleed stage, interventional radiology may be helpful.

- Otherwise:
  - First, be aware of the patient's resuscitation status!
  - Apply a lot of pressure to the bleeding point.
  - Get senior help.
  - Get to theatre.
  - Resuscitate as best you can whilst on the way to theatre.
  - The only chance of survival (~10%) is prompt arrest of bleeding.
  - Ischaemic stroke is a recognized complication of surgery, but the alternative to surgery is death.
- In some scenarios the patient should not be actively managed, and may have specifically requested not to be resuscitated or returned to theatre. This is the usually the case in patients who have incurable cancer and are aware of the risk of death from carotid blow-out.
- There will be a carotid blow-out protocol to hand. Everything will be well documented and managed by head and neck nurses and the palliative care team. This situation calls for calmness and peace, as best as can be achieved for the patient and their relatives. Read the protocol and discuss with the palliative care team about it if you ever have any patients in this category on your ward. Most protocols include the use of diamorphine and midazolam. Letting someone go can be one of the hardest things for a doctor to do, but you will be better for it. It is always traumatic for everyone because of the horrendous nature of the event, and don't feel bad if you are struggling to cope emotionally after such a case—there is always help at hand via the occupational health department.

Retrobulbar haemorrhage

General points

- Bleeding behind the eye can follow trauma to the periorbital region or after surgery such as orbital floor repair, reduction of fractured zygoma, or obviously ophthalmic surgery. The incidence is 0.3% of these fractures or following surgery for them.
- The pathophysiology is complicated, but for simplicity think of it as a type of compartment syndrome where bleeding occurs in the orbit causing a rise in intra-orbital pressure which leads to blindness by ischaemic injury to the anterior optic nerve.
- Primary treatment is increase the volume of orbit and to a lesser extent try to reduce the pressures in the orbit medically.
- Prompt decompression <90min from the onset of symptoms will save sight. Delay, usually due to failure to recognize RBH (by not looking for it), leads to blindness.

How to recognize RBH

- In a trauma or postoperative patient reducing visual acuity plus any one of the following must be considered to be RBH:
  - pain
  - proptosis
  - ophthalmoplegia
  - loss of direct light reflex (with preservation of consensual reflex for distinction candidates)
  - tense hard eye.

Management of RBH (Fig. 10.3)

- The diagnosis is clinical. Imaging should not delay treatment
- Treatment is surgical ± medical
- Call your senior, but you may be expected to perform the decompression. Time is of the essence
- If you are taking a phone call about a patient in an ED at another hospital, you should advise them to get someone to do a decompression (senior ED doctor or ophthalmologist), or to start the medical management in the meantime and prepare to transfer the patient to you if no one is available to manage the surgical decompression
- If your senior will be there soon, he may advise you to start the medical management and prepare equipment for decompression

Surgical decompression of RBH

- If you are with the patient, perform a lateral canthotomy and inferior cantholysis immediately. There is no need to go to theatre.
  - Inject LA around the lateral canthus.
  - Take an artery clip and crush the lateral canthus between the jaws all the way from the junction of the upper and lower lids down to the orbital rim.
  - Cut the crushed tissue with scissors. this will allow the lower eyelid to swing out.

Algorithm of the Management Options for a Retrobulbar Hemorrhage

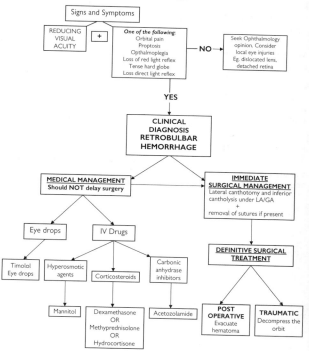

Fig. 10.3 Algorithm of the management options for a retrobulbar haemorrhage. Reproduced from *Journal of Oral and Maxillofacial Surgery*, **65**: 2, Winterton *et al.*, Review of management options for a retrobulbar hemorrhage. Copyright (2007), with permission from Elsevier.

- Now locate the inferior canthus with the tips of the scissors and cut it.
- When you release the tense inferior canthus, the orbital septum and the proptosed globe will pop forwards.
- Keep cutting the canthus until this has happened. Don't be afraid. There is no tissue there that you are cutting which cannot be repaired at a later date, but loss of vision is permanent!
- Now monitor. If visual acuity is returning over a few minutes—great.
- If not, you either need more surgery or it may be that that medical management in combination with surgery is required, and your senior

will have to decide whether more decompression is possible or whether to start some drugs.

- Following this immediate management, the patient needs to be prepared for definitive surgery in theatre under GA. This may include evacuation of a clot if postoperative or further decompression if post-trauma.

Medical management of RBH

- Acetazolamide is a carbonic anhydrase inhibitor and shrinks the vitreous but has a delayed effect. Give 500mg IV.
- Mannitol is an osmotic diuretic and has an immediate effect. Give 20ml of 20% mannitol IV quickly.
- Hydrocortisone 100mg IV may also be of benefit.
- Megadoses of corticosteroids are unproven in RBH and are probably dangerous.

Final point on RBH

When you are called to see a patient with pan-facial fractures who is already intubated, you should consider possibility that they have a RBH and the clock started ticking from time of the injury.

Commonly used drugs and dental materials

Local anaesthetics

Getting good anaesthesia is the key to stress-free procedures.

- The administration technique may be more important than product selection (📖 see p. 190), but you should be well informed about the drug you are using.
- LA used for dental administration is typically of higher concentration than that used for non-dental reasons in order to limit the volume. Vasoconstrictor reduces the dose further; without it the duration of action may be too short.
- LA is presented in 1.8ml or 2.2ml cartridges compatible with dental syringes and can be used outside the oral cavity except in extremities such as the nose tip and ear. Although some surgeons will disagree with this it is safer to avoid vasoconstrictors in extremites.

Safe dosages

- A rough estimate of one cartridge of 2% solution per 10kg body weight will keep you well below the toxic dose.
- This should give sufficient anaesthesia in most cases. If not think about reasons for failure.
- If two cartridges have not had sufficient effect, consider using a different preparation.
- For children, a rule of thumb is 1–2 cartridges in under-fives, up to 3 cartridges for under-tens, and 4 cartridges for children >10 years, although manufacturers recommend that the dose is calculated by weight for each child.

Preparations

The commonly used injectable preparations are shown in Table 11.1. In practice 2% lidocaine with 1:80,000 adrenaline is the most widely used solution. However, bupivacaine and articaine can be very effective where longer-lasting anaesthesia is required. There have been reports of neuro-toxicity using these higher-concentration solutions, so nerve block is not recommended.

Toxicity

- The most common cause of toxicity is inadvertent IV injection so always aspirate first. Signs include:
  - disturbed taste, circum-oral tingling (not reliable signs in our patients!), confusion, dizziness, drowsiness, and fitting.
  - Arrhythmia with ↑/↓ BP depending on whether adrenaline has been used.
- Management is airway maintenance and control of fitting until the effect of the LA has worn off.

Table 11.1 Commonly used dental local anaesthetics

	Lidocaine	Articaine	Mepivacaine	Prilocaine
Trade name	Xylocaine® Lignospan Special®	Septocaine® Septanest®	Scandonest L®	Citanest®
Concentration	1% 2%	4%	2% 3% (plain)	3% 4% (plain)
Vasoconstrictor	1:80,000 adrenaline	1:100,000 or 1:200,000 adrenaline	1:200,000 adrenaline 1:20,000 levonordefrin	1:1,850,00 Felypressin (Octapressin®)
Maximum recommended dose (with vasoconstrictor)	7mg/kg (11 cartridges for 70kg adult)	7mg/kg	7mg/kg	8mg/kg <10ml recommended
Duration of action (with vasoconstrictor)	45min	60min	60–100min	45min
❶		Neurotoxicity possible. Avoid using for nerve block		Methaemo-globinaemia reported in overdose Avoid in pregnancy

Allergy

Allergy to LA is extremely rare. The allergen may be:
- preservative (eg. metabisulphite) in which case preservative-free preparations are available
- latex used in the rubber bung.

Most patients who have a bad experience with LA have done so because it is not properly administered or for psychological reasons.[1]

1 Rood JP (2000). *British Dental Journal* **189**; 380–4.

Analgesics and sedatives

Dental pain can be excruciating—think of Tom Hanks self-extracting a tooth in the film *Castaway*. In contrast, pain is often well tolerated in patients with facial fractures and after facial surgery. Discomfort from postoperative swelling may be improved by early use of steroids.

Sustained tooth pain, irreversible pulpitis, will require some sort of procedure to remove the infected tissue, either root canal therapy or extraction of the tooth. Likewise, abscesses will usually require surgical intervention.

Achieving good anaesthesia during procedures such as surgical extraction will reduce postoperative analgesic requirements. Long-acting anaesthetics such as Marcaine® are recommended for this reason.

There are a few pain conditions affecting the head, such as trigeminal neuralgia, which require specialized treatment (see p. 128).

Topical analgesics

- Lidocaine 5%–benzocaine 20% ointment—apply to the buccal sulcus for 2–3min before injecting LA (see p. 190).
- Benzydamine mouth rinse can be used for painful ulcerative conditions and radiation mucositis (see pp. 137, 218).
- Benzocaine lozenges are also useful for the above conditions.

Oral analgesics

- NSAIDs have been shown to be effective as both analgesics and anti-inflammatories following dento-alveolar surgery.
- Ibuprofen is an excellent postoperative analgesic for simple and surgical extractions. Up to 400mg qds is regularly prescribed for pain.
- Paracetamol—studies have shown paracetamol to be effective after surgical wisdom tooth removal. Combine with ibuprofen for better effect.
- Diclofenac sodium—50mg tds PO or PR is useful after major surgery.
- Opiates—patients undergoing major surgery should have PRN morphate sulphate solution considered. Co-codamol 30/500 or dihydrocodeine are commonly prescribed postoperatively.
- Carbamazepine—this is not an analgesic but nonetheless is used to control pain in trigeminal neuralgia. 300mg tds is increased up to a maximum of 2.4g or until analgesia is achieved.
- Tricyclic and other selective antidepressants such as fluoxetine have an important role in the management of AFP.

Sedatives

- Diazepam—dental anxiety is not uncommon and some patients may require a small dose of benzodiazepine as pre-procedure anxiolysis. Diazepam 5mg the night before and on the morning of the appointment will produce a mild sedative effect. Patients will require an escort and should not drive if this regime is used.

- Alternatively, temazepam, a shorter-acting drug, can be given 1 hour pre-surgery at a dose of 10–30mg, depending on weight, alcohol tolerance, and effect.
- Midazolam—this is the drug of choice for operator-controlled conscious sedation. It gives an excellent anxiolytic and amnesic effect but is not analgesic so LA must also be used.
  - Check that the patient has an escort before starting.
  - Check medical history and consent.
  - Check that a suitably trained assistant is available (specialist sedation trained nurses).
  - Pulse oximetry is mandatory throughout. BP must be checked before starting.
  - Site cannula in forearm. Give 2mg bolus over 90sec (halve this for elderly patients).
  - Wait for 90sec before giving further 1mg boluses until adequate sedation is achieved (patient should be drowsy but able to follow commands). It is unusual to need more than 10mg.
  - Further boluses can be given during the procedure.
  - The patient must stay in the department until a trained staff member deems that they have fully recovered by.
  - You must have the reversal agent (flumazenil) available when using midazolam, but be aware that it has a shorter half-life than midazolam and administration may need to be repeated.
- Nitrous oxide (N_2O)—inhalational sedation is widely used in dentistry, particularly paediatric dentistry. N_2O is delivered via a nasal mask to produce relative analgesia. Local anaesthetic must still be used.
  - Check consent, and that escort and assistant are available.
  - Contraindicated in nasal obstruction and first trimester of pregnancy.
  - Start with 100% O_2. Add 10% N_2O for 1min and then increase to 20% for 1min. Increase N_2O by 5% every minute until adequately sedated (usual range 20–50%).
  - Recover with 100% O_2 and slowly raise up to sitting.
  - N_2O may cause circum-oral paraesthesia and is a drug open to abuse! Long-term exposure can cause a wide range of neurological effects.

Antimicrobials

- Odontogenic infections are polymicrobial and often anaerobic. Penicillins are still often effective.
- Latest NICE guidelines (http://guidance.nice.org.uk/CG64) state that antibiotic prophylaxis against endocarditis during dental procedures is not indicated.
- Antibiotics should not be a substitute for pulp extirpation, tooth extraction, or pus drainage.
- In severe infections where the airway is or could become compromised, antibiotics are *definitely not* a substitute (📖 see pp. 98, 233).

Antibacterial

The indications for commonly used antibiotics are listed below. Where possible swabs should be taken for sensitivity before starting, but in the mouth causative organisms can be difficult to isolate from normal oral flora.

- Amoxicillin—500mg tds for standard postoperative prophylaxis (e.g. after oro-antral communication). Up to 500mg tds in oral infections. Co-amoxiclav 375mg tds is also a good choice.
- Metronidazole—400mg tds orally/500mg tds IV. Combine with a penicillin for dental infection or after fracture communicating with the mouth or sinuses (alveolar fractures are open fractures). Beware warfarin.
- Benzylpenicillin—IV penicillin for dental infections and fractures.
- Erythromycin—used for penicillin-allergic patients.
- Clindamycin—for osteomyelitis.
- Chlorhexidine 0.2% mouthwash—effective for general disinfection of the mouth. Part of the standard postoperative protocol when intra-oral wounds have been made. It is not a substitute for tooth brushing. Long-term use can cause reversible staining of teeth.
- Tetracycline—avoid using this in children under 12 at it causes permanent staining of the teeth.
- Flucloxacillin—250–500mg qds for skin/soft tissue infections.

Antifungal

Oral candidal infection is common, particularly in the very young, the elderly, denture wearers, the immunocompromised, and the malnourished. As this is a large proportion of hospital inpatients, *Candida* should be at the top of your list when reviewing patients with sore mouths (📖 see p. 216). Remembering a small list of drugs will be a great help.

- Nystatin suspension—100,000 units (1ml) held in mouth qds.
- Miconazole gel 2%—apply 5–10ml qds to oral mucosa after meals.
- Fluconazole—50mg capsules once daily for severe infections (+ topical treatment).

Antiviral

Primary HSV infection (herpetic gingivostomatits) can be extremely painful and the patient (usually a child) may be quite unwell. Herpes zoster reactivation as shingles, particularly when affecting the ophthalmic division of the CN V or causing CN VII palsy (Ramsay Hunt syndrome) also requires prompt treatment.

- Aciclovir 200mg PO five times daily (can be increased in severe cases). Child is half adult dose. Topical treatment is available for herpes labialis (cold sore)—aciclovir cream (5% aciclovir).
- If the ophthalmic division of trigeminal nerve is affected, request an ophthalmology opinion, as associated dendritic corneal ulceration can cause lasting damage if not seen and treated early.
- Scottish Dental Clinical Effectiveness Programme has useful guidelines for prescribing for common dental conditions (www.sdcep.org.uk).

Dental materials

The dental armamentarium contains hundreds of materials with new products constantly appearing. A few materials are regularly used in OMFS practice.

- ▶ Get someone to show you where the materials are kept and how to mix/apply them **before** you need to use them
- ▶ Dentists in practice do not work alone and neither should you. Get someone to assist you

Some useful materials are listed below.

Dressings

- Ledermix®—corticosteriod–antibiotic dressing paste applied directly to inflamed pulps. Particularly useful where LA is ineffective due to infection. Cover over with a temporary filling material and prescribe anti-biotics if indicated.
- Alvogyl®– fibrous dressing used to pack a dry socket (📖 see p. 195). Its effects are antimicrobial and analgesic. Do not decontaminate the whole pot by using a dirty instrument to dispense some.
- Whitehead's varnish—iodoform-based resin that is used to pack large cavities (e.g after bone cyst removal). The dressing is antiseptic and can be changed at regular intervals to check healing.

Temporary filling materials

- There are a number of zinc oxide and eugenol-based materials such as IRM®, Kalzinol®, and Cavit®.
- They come as a paste and powder which are mixed before use.
- You should be able to form a firm 'sausage' which you can roll between your fingers before packing it in the tooth. Press down with a damp cotton roll or pledget to condense.
- Can last for up to 2 weeks.

Filling and bonding materials

Composite

- Tooth-coloured filling material which is useful for splinting teeth (📖 see p. 199). It comes in a variety of shades in premixed tubes.
- The tooth is prepared with an acid etch and bonding agent for a strong bond to form but this may be omitted if it is just a temporary measure.
- Composite is sensitive to water contamination, so the tooth must be dry. Use cotton rolls to keep tongue and cheeks away.
- Command set is activated by blue light (don't forget to protect eyes) which polymerizes the material hard within 40sec.

Glass ionomer cement (GIC)

- Tooth-coloured filling material. It comes as a powder and liquid for hand mixing or in capsule that needs high-speed mixing.
- A useful material for retrograde filling of a root canal in apicectomy and for cementing appliances to teeth.

Dental amalgam

Watch out for the following.

- Amalgam tattoo—inadvertent implantation into mucosa. May be confused with a pigmented lesion (📖 see p. 222).
- Lichenoid reaction – white patches on the mucosa adjacent to the filling (📖 see p. 220).
- Streak artefacts—shine from the metal can make interpretation of CT difficult.
- Inadvertent damage to a large amalgam restoration in the tooth adjacent to your extraction. Cover over with a temporary filling material and ask the GDP to replace.
- Mercury poisoning—there is no evidence that mercury released from amalgam fillings causes systemic illness. BDA guidelines state that amalgam is safe to use and that sound fillings should not be removed. ✒ (http://www.bda.org/dentists/policy-research/bda-policies/public-health/fact-files/amalgam.aspx).

Impression materials

For technique 📖 see p. 207.

- Alginate—seaweed-derived hydrocolloid which does not taste unpleasant and is easy to work with. Accuracy is not as good as that of other materials. The powder is mixed with tapwater. Working time is short so move quickly. Alginate will dry out and deform, so it must be wrapped in damp paper towels and sent to the laboratory straight away to be poured up as a plaster model (ideally within 1 hour).
- Elastomers—these can be polyethers, polysulphides, or silicones. They are very accurate, so they are used to construct close-fitting appliances such as obturators. This can also make them difficult to remove from the mouth! They are quite stable and so do not need to be poured immediately (store dry). They are usually premixed and machine dispensed. Some are retarded by latex, so check first before handling with gloved hands.

Miscellaneous

- Gutta percha—naturally occurring radio-opaque rubber, which is used to fill the canal space after root canal therapy. Gutta percha is produced as very fine points and is ideally suited to inserting into a sinus tract to locate its origin radiographically.
- Coe-Pak®—a periodontal dressing which is used to protect healing tissue or for splinting. Mixed from two tubes of paste, you must use petroleum jelly on your gloves and patient's lips before handling otherwise it will stick where you don't want it to!

People with whom you will be working

Other surgeons

ENT surgeons

- ENT surgeons are probably our closest colleagues and you will often find that we share wards, junior doctors, clinics, and also patients.
- There are many occasions in OMFS when you will work with ENT surgeons and you will usually find the relationship mutually beneficial.
- ENT surgeons are members of the head and neck MDT.
- You may be asked to see ENT cases with head and neck abscesses on the ward to give an opinion, often to see whether the abscess has a dental origin. The arrangement is, of course, reciprocal.
- ENT surgeons are occasionally asked to employ their endoscopic sinus skills to help with retrieval of tooth roots or implants from the sinuses, or even to reduce orbital floor fractures or to decompress RBH.
- Some TMJ patients first present to the ENT with ear ache.

Plastic surgeons

- Plastic surgeons are also usually members of the head and neck MDT.
- In most OMFS units the OMFS surgeons do their own reconstruction, including microvascular free flaps. However, ENT surgeons often call upon plastic surgeons to work with them as the reconstructive team, and OMFS surgeons do so occasionally.
- You may find that the ED will have some arrangement with the local plastic and OMFS teams regarding the management of facial lacerations, and you should be aware what this is.

Ophthalmic surgeons

- You will often call upon the help of the ophthalmic team mainly for the management of trauma patients with periorbital and zygomatic complex fractures. These patients may or may not have globe injuries (see p. 72).
- Ophthalmic surgeons are also often involved in the management of periorbital cancer resections and also problems such as entropion, ectropion, and dacrorhinosinusitis.
- A sub-specialty is oculoplastic surgery. Oculoplastic surgeons are highly skilled at managing eyelid problems such as BCC, SCC, and other pathology in and around the lids. It is usually sensible to seek an opinion in such cases or transfer the patient to their care.

Dental specialists

General practice dentists

- Otherwise known as dental surgeons or general dental practitioners.
- Most of their referrals to OMFS units are from GDPs.
- By far the most frequent referral a GDP makes to a district general hospital is to the OMFS department.
- You may also find that a GDP calls you to make an emergency referral about something you may not consider an emergency—a common example is a failed extraction.
- Whilst you have to fulfil your priorities with your experiences as a hospital doctor, you should try to be aware that the GDP does not have the hospital resources that you have to hand. Until you have worked in the community setting you may not appreciate how difficult it is to deal with complications outside of a hospital. Therefore you should try to show some empathy and help as best you can—they may also be friendly with the consultant and give you either positive or negative feedback!

Periodontists

- Periodontists deal with the tissues supporting the teeth, i.e. the gingivae, periodontal ligament, cementum, and alveolar bone.
- In practice this means that they deal with periodontal pocketing and dental implantology (numerous people deal with dental implants).
- They are encountered mainly either in the primary care setting (not NHS) or in dental hospitals.

Endodontists

- Endodontists deal with root canal treatment and apical surgery.
- Developments in root canal therapy have radically reduced the numbers of patients who require apicectomy and this is an improvement in patient care.
- Endodontists also provide apical surgery under magnification, which gives much better results.
- However, like periodontists, they are not generally available on the NHS outside dental hospitals.

Orthodontists

- Orthodontists are the dental specialist you are most likely to encounter in a district general hospital. This is because of their role in childrens' dental care.
- Hospital-based orthodontists usually deal with children with severely crowded teeth and are also part of the cleft palate team.
- Hospital based orthodontists are a part of the orthognathic team (see p. 142).
- Community-based orthodontists usually provide a mixture of private and NHS practice in accordance with NHS guidelines on what the NHS will pay for.

Paediatric dentists

- Paediatric dentists are not generally available on the high street but are available in community centres, teaching hospitals, dental schools, and some specialist units. They are part of the cleft palate team.

Oral surgeons

- Oral surgeons are employed almost exclusively in dental schools and are involved in surgery of the structures which support the teeth and oral tissues. However, times are changing, and there is a move to employ oral surgeons in the district general hospital setting as well.
- They are also involved in dental implants and bone grafting to the jaws.
- There are many staff grade and associate specialists (collectively termed SAS) in OMFS unit who are on the specialist GDC list for oral surgery. These practitioners are not the same as consultant oral surgeons who have completed specialist training just like other consultants.
- Some consultant oral surgeons may have been appointed based on previous experience/training (grandfathering). There are now several training schemes and a Specialty Advisory Committee (SAC) in oral surgery.

Restorative dentist

- Restorative dentists are not usually available outside dental schools or private care, except as part of the head and neck MDT.
- In the MDT they provide an opinion about which teeth need to be extracted prior to radiotherapy fields which may involve the jaws. They can also advise and help with dentures, dental implants, and dental obturators (for maxillectomy patients).
- In dental schools and private practice their practice is mainly concerned with crown and bridge work, inlays, and veneers.

Prosthodontists

- Prosthodontists are experts on fixed or removable false teeth.
- In private practice this means removable false teeth or dentures and bridges, with or without dental implants. They may also be part of the head and neck MDT instead of a restorative dentist.

Members of the multidisciplinary head and neck team

General points

- This list is not intended to be exhaustive and there is some variation between units
- There will be no repetition of plastic surgeons, ENT surgeons, or restorative dentists and prosthodontists as these are noted in the previous section.

The histopathologist

- The head and neck histopathologist may be a dental pathologist who may or may not also have a medical degree, but more commonly is a medically qualified histopathologist. Either way they are highly skilled experts on oral pathology and without them OMFS is very much more difficult.
- They are key to the success of head and neck MDTs.
- If your district general hospital does not have a dedicated oral or head and neck histopathologist, you may find that some of the unusual pathologies that you see, especially rare salivary gland lesions, will be forwarded to oral pathologists.
- When a diagnosis of lymphoma has been made, the case is often reviewed by a designated lymphoma expert/panel who may not be the same person as the head and neck pathologist.

The clinical oncologist

- Head and neck clinical oncologists are often the 'bridge' within the MDT that unites the ENT and OMF surgeons.
- They oversee chemo- and radiotherapy. As non-surgeons, they often have a different perspective and their input is invaluable.

The radiologist

- Head and neck radiologists are responsible to the MDT for reporting on the staging scans.
- They also work alongside the oncologists to plan radiotherapy.
- They will be available in the one-stop neck lump clinic where they provide ultrasound expertise.
- Interventional radiologists will oversee investigations such as angio-graphy, and CT or MR angiography.

Speech and language therapist (SALT)

- The SALT should see all the head and neck cancer patients prior to treatment (surgical or medical) and will be called upon to help with post-treatment rehabilitation.
- They are particularly useful for assessing both speech and swallowing function post-surgery. They will see patients with the radiologist and discuss barium swallows. They also have input in patients with aspiration following treatment and in assessing whether patients can eat/drink safely.
- Many are often actively involved in research.

The dietician

- The dietician should see all head and neck cancer patients pre-operatively.
- Often they will liaise with the PEG, RIG, or even TPN service.
- Postoperatively they oversee the patient's nutrition through oral, PEG, NG, or parenteral routes.
- They will provide help if your patient has special needs such as those with chyle leaks who need medium-chain triglyceride diets.

The clinical nurse specialist

- Clinical nurse specialist are key workers for head and neck cancer patients. They liaise with the other specialists and feed back to the consultant team
- They provide emotional and practical support, and as such are highly skilled in a wide range of medical and psychological disciplines

The research nurse

- Research nurses are highly prized members of MDTs.
- They are involved in patient recruitment and day-to-day management of patients in trials and data collection.

Palliative care consultant

- Palliative care consultants are increasingly involved in MDTs.
- It is widely acknowledges that a significant number of cases discussed at the MDT are not at a stage where curative treatment is an option, and many of these patients benefit from palliative care specialists.
- Quality of death or dying is rarely considered, but is very important for those patients with endstage disease.[1]

1 Ethunandan M, Hoffman G, Morey PJ, Brennan PA (2005). *Oral Surgery, Oral Medicine, Oral Pathology, Oral Radiology, and Endodontics* **100**: 147–52.

Eponyms and maxillofacial syndromes

Apert syndrome is a craniosynostosis plus syndactyly leading to lack of anterior growth of the midface, raised intracranial pressure, and blindness due subluxation and lack of corneal cover of the eye.

Behçet syndrome is a multisystem autoimmune condition associated with HLA-B5. Patients have oral and genital ulceration and uveitis. Treatment is highly specialized; mainly immunosuppressant.

Binder syndrome Patients have severe under-development of the nose and maxilla.

Cleidocranial dysostosis is a condition mainly of membranous bone formation leading to hypoplastic or aplastic clavicles, and frontal and parietal bossing on a large but shortened skull with midface retrusion, clefting, and failure of tooth eruption common.

Crouzon syndrome These patients have craniosynostosis and a hypo-plastic midface which may lead to blindness. The increased intracranial pressure will lead to mental retardation, if left untreated.

DiGeorge syndrome is a combination of cardiac anomalies, velopharyngeal anomalies, thymic aplasia, and hypocalcaemia. It is due to deletion of part of chromosome 22.

Eagle syndrome is a painful condition due to elongation of the styloid process which causes pain on turning the head.

Ehlers–Danlos syndrome involves a group of inherited connective tissue disorders resulting in, amongst other things, hyperflexibility of joints, increased bleeding sometimes, possibly more TMJ problems, highly elastic skin, etc.

Frey syndrome Gustatory sweating after parotid surgery. A similar thing can happen with running nose after nasal surgery and sweating over the face after submandibular surgery.

Gardner syndrome is familial colorectal polyposis plus craniofacial osteomas, epidermoid cysts, and fibromas of skin.

Goldenhar syndrome is a syndrome of first and second branchial arch anomalies with hemifacial microsomia and other anomalies of the internal organs.

Gorlin–Goltz syndrome, or multiple basal cell naevi syndrome. Sufferers from this condition have multiple BCCs, keratocystic odontogenic tumours, bifid ribs, and calcification of the falx cerebri.

Heerfordt syndrome results from sarcoidosis affecting the parotid and lacrimal glands with facial nerve weakness and fever.

Histiocytosis X is the general term for group of syndromes involving histiocytes.
- Langerhans cell histiocytosis, which is also called histiocytosis X. This has three groups.
  - Solitary eosinophilic granuloma—may affect the mandible.
  - Hand–Schuller–Christian disease—multifocal and affects younger children. Treatment is cytotoxic.
  - Letterer–Siwe disease is generalized and often rapidly fatal.

- Malignant histiocytosis syndrome (now known as T-cell lymphoma).
- Non-Langerhans cell histiocytosis (also known as haemophagocytic syndrome).

Horner syndrome is a combination of miosis, ptosis, anhydrosis, and enopthalmos. It is due to ipsilateral sympathetic dysfunction such as iatrogenic, after neck surgery, or lung cancer.

Hurler syndrome or mucopolysaccharidosis type 1. It consists of hepatosplenomegaly, dwarfism, frontal bossing, enlarged tongue, coarse features, and mental retardation.

Larsen syndrome is an autosomal dominant congenital disorder. comprising cleft palate, with other anomalies including hypermobility and brachycephaly.

MAGIC syndrome involves mouth and genital ulcers and interstitial chondritis. It seems to overlap Behçet syndrome and relapsing poly-chondritis.

Marcus Gunn phenomenon or trigemino-oculomotor synkinesis. This is an inherited condition of eyelid retraction on moving the jaw.

Marfan syndrome is a disorder of connective tissue which results in aortic root dilatation, long limbs and digits, high arch palate, and tall thin stature. It is common in basket-ball players.

McCune–Albright syndrome is a combination of polyostotic fibrous dysplasia, café au lait spots, and endocrine anomaly, which is most commonly precocious puberty.

Melkerson–Rosenthal syndrome comprises facial nerve weakness, fissured tongue, and facial swelling. It is a type of orofacial granuloma-tosis.

Paterson–Brown–Kelly syndrome or **Plummer–Vinson syndrome** comprises anaemia, post-cricoid webbing, and dysphagia which usually affects middle-aged women. There is a dangerous tendency to develop cancer in the webbed area.

Peutz–Jeughers syndrome results in intestinal polyps, with peri-oral and intra-oral pigmentation. The polyps are hamartomas and are not pre-maliganant.

Ramsay Hunt syndrome type 2 is one of three syndromes named after Ramsay Hunt. It is the other non-iatrogneic cause of lower facial nerve weakness (other than Bell's palsy and tumour) that you are most likely to encounter and is otherwise known as herpes zoster osicus. It is the result of herpes zoster infection of the of geniculate ganglion, causing ipsilateral facial nerve palsy and vesicles in the external auditory canal.

Robin sequence, or **Pierre–Robin sequence** is a congenital condition resulting in a severely small lower jaw, cleft palate, and glossoptosis. It can be fatal if the tongue is not prevented from obstructing the airway.

Romberg syndrome or **Parry–Romberg syndrome** is a rare disfiguring disease with progressive hemifacial atrophy, wasting of the soft tissues of the face, epilepsy, and trigeminal neuralgia. It tends to burn out after a few years, but leaves a facial asymmetry which is very difficult to treat. It is of unknown aetiology.

Sjögren's syndrome
- Primary Sjögren's syndrome or sicca syndrome is dry mouth and eyes.
- Secondary Sjögren's syndrome is as primary plus another autoimmune disease such as rheumatoid arthritis, systemic lupus erythematosus.

Stevens–Johnson syndrome is a type of toxic epidermal necrolysis. It is an autoimmune condition usually triggered by an exogenous agent such as herpesvirus or one of many drugs. It results in ulceration of the oral, genital, anal, and conjunctival membranes, and also affects the skin. A milder form is erythema multiforme.

Stickler syndrome is a connective tissue disorder which results in a flat face, cleft palate, myopia, cataracts, hearing loss, arthritis, and hypermobility.

Sturge–Weber syndrome comprises a large port wine stain of the upper face, epilepsy, mental retardation, and glaucoma.

Treacher Collins syndrome or mandibulo-facial dysostosis comprises under-development of the mandible, zygoma, and ears with a downward-sloping palpebral fissure.

Trotter syndrome is a combination of symptoms of malignancy invading the infratemporal fossa and lateral pharynx and includes pain in the mandibular division of the trigeminal nerve, trismus and immobility of palate, and unilateral conductive hearing loss. It is possible that TMJ pain could be confused with this condition and vice versa.

von Recklinghausen neurofibromatosis includes neurofibromas with premalignant potential, café au lait spots, and skeletal anomalies.

Index